Rym Maamouri

Ocular sarcoidosis

Rym Maamouri

Ocular sarcoidosis

clinical study and diagnostic orientation

ScienciaScripts

Imprint

Any brand names and product names mentioned in this book are subject to trademark, brand or patent protection and are trademarks or registered trademarks of their respective holders. The use of brand names, product names, common names, trade names, product descriptions etc. even without a particular marking in this work is in no way to be construed to mean that such names may be regarded as unrestricted in respect of trademark and brand protection legislation and could thus be used by anyone.

Cover image: www.ingimage.com

This book is a translation from the original published under ISBN 978-620-3-45906-7.

Publisher:
Sciencia Scripts
is a trademark of
Dodo Books Indian Ocean Ltd. and OmniScriptum S.R.L publishing group

120 High Road, East Finchley, London, N2 9ED, United Kingdom
Str. Armeneasca 28/1, office 1, Chisinau MD-2012, Republic of Moldova, Europe
Printed at: see last page
ISBN: 978-620-6-28767-4

Abstract

Introduction

Sarcoidosis is a multi-systemic inflammatory disease of unknown etiology, characterized by the presence of granulomas without caseous necrosis. Ocular involvement accounts for 11.8% of uveitis cases. Our aim is to study the clinical and epidemiological characteristics of patients with sarcoidosis uveitis.

Patients and Methods

This is a 6-year retrospective study of 9 patients with sarcoidosis in an ophthalmology department. All our patients benefited from a complete ophthalmological examination combined with multimodal imaging and complementary examinations for diagnostic and prognostic purposes.

Results

We included 9 patients (8 women and 1 man). Of the 9 patients, 4 presented with initial ocular manifestations revealing systemic involvement, while the diagnosis of systemic sarcoidosis preceded ocular involvement in 5 patients. Sarcoidosis uveitis was found in 100% of patients; the mean age at first consultation was 49 years (29-58). Ophthalmological involvement was bilateral in all patients and not always symmetrical. 2 patients (22%) had anterior uveitis, 1 (11%) patient had intermediate uveitis, 2 patients (22%) had both anterior and intermediate uveitis and 4 patients (44%) had posterior involvement which was classified as panuveitis with retinal vasculitis in 1 case, panuveitis with multifocal choroiditis in 2 cases and panuveitis with retinal vasculitis and multifocal choroiditis in 1 case.Treatment was based mainly on topical corticoids alone (2 patients) or combined with oral corticoids (7 patients). Progression was favorable under treatment.

Discussion

Our results are in line with those reported in the literature. Our series reveals a female predominance and uveitis as the most frequent ocular manifestation. Sarcoidosis uveitis is generally bilateral and may be anterior (35-60% of cases), intermediate (6-10% of cases) or posterior (14-43% of cases).

Diagnosis is based on a range of clinical and paraclinical arguments, both ocular and systemic. Treatment is based on topical and oral corticosteroids, with immunosuppressive agents as second-line therapy.

Conclusion

Ocular involvement in sarcoidosis is frequent and can be revelatory of the disease. Bilateral granulomatous uveitis, intermediate uveitis or panuveitis should be investigated. Its management is multidisciplinary, involving both ophthalmologists and internists, in order to improve its prognosis.

1. Introduction

Sarcoidosis is a chronic inflammatory disease of unknown origin, characterized by the presence of systemic non-caseating granulomas in the lungs, skin, lymph nodes, heart, liver, eyes and other areas.

[1] The eye is the second most affected organ in sarcoidosis, after the lungs [2]. Being a highly sensitive sensory organ, ocular symptoms prompt patients to consult an ophthalmologist at an early stage. Ophthalmologists therefore have an important role to play in the early diagnosis of sarcoidosis through ophthalmological examinations and systemic assessments.

Around 30-50% of sarcoidosis patients develop intraocular inflammation known as uveitis [2-3]. This inflammation may be isolated, with no systemic involvement.

Sarcoidosis can also affect different parts of the eye and adjacent tissues, leading to uveitis, episcleritis/scleritis, eyelid abnormalities, conjunctival granuloma, optic neuropathy, lacrimal gland enlargement and orbital inflammation.

Complications of inflammation or treatment side-effects can also include the development of glaucoma and cataracts. Ocular manifestations may occur in isolation, or may be associated with involvement of other organs. Ocular sarcoidosis can manifest itself in a variety of ways and present different degrees of severity in patients. A multidisciplinary approach is required to achieve the best treatment outcomes for both ocular and systemic manifestations.

Sarcoidosis can affect virtually any structure in the eye, as well as surrounding tissues. In many cases, sarcoidosis initially manifests as ocular symptoms. It is essential that ophthalmologists and physicians in other specialties are aware of the variety of ocular manifestations associated with sarcoidosis.

2. Epidemiology

Data on ocular sarcoidosis in African-Americans are limited, but these patients appear to present ophthalmologically with uveitis and/or adnexal granuloma at a younger age than Caucasian patients [4]. Uveitis remains the most common ocular pathology outside Sicca's syndrome [5]. The prevalence of sarcoidosis in a population of uveitis patients varies according to factors such as age, gender, ethnic origin, diagnostic methods used (e.g. positron emission tomography) and the type of patient recruitment (tertiary care center or not) [4,6,7]. In tertiary care centers, the incidence of sarcoidosis ranges from 0.48 to 11.4 cases per 100,000 people per year worldwide [8]. A higher incidence is observed in African-Americans, reaching 17.8 cases per 100,000 people per year [9,10]. The prevalence of ocular sarcoidosis ranges from 10% to 50% in studies of Caucasian populations [11,12]. In contrast, ocular sarcoidosis is more common in the Asian population, particularly in Japan, where it has become the leading cause of uveitis, accounting for around 15% of all cases [13,14] ;

The prevalence of ocular involvement varies according to the series studied, ranging from *13%* (Turkish study) to 79% (Japanese study) of patients with systemic sarcoidosis. [15,16]. In approximately 20-30% of patients [17,18]. Ocular involvement is the main symptom. Uveitis is present in 30-70% of cases, and remains the most frequent ocular pathology apart from Sicca syndrome [5]. Conjunctival nodules are found in 40% of cases. [15]. A study of 121 patients with sarcoidosis revealed that men (56%) were more likely to develop ocular involvement than women (23%)[18].

Sarcoidosis can also affect children, with most cases occurring between the ages of 8 and 15. [19]. However, some patients diagnosed early with sarcoidosis are now recognized as having Blau syndrome with de novo genetic mutations. [20]. The distribution of ocular involvement in adults shows a peak incidence between the ages of 20 and 30, and another between the ages of 50 and 60. [15]. The average age of presentation of uveitis is 42 years, with a wide variability ranging from 4 to 82 years. [20]. African-Americans with sarcoidosis are more likely to develop ocular involvement than Caucasians. [22]. In addition, race may influence the age of onset of uveitis, with blacks tending to develop it between the ages of 35 and 44, while whites show a peak incidence between the ages of 43 and 52. [21,23].

In specialized centers, sarcoidosis accounts for around 1-3% of uveitis cases in children [24,25]. Whereas it is associated with around 10% of uveitis cases in adults. [26,27]. An epidemiological study conducted in the southeastern United States revealed that sarcoidosis was the cause of uveitis in 11% of the study population, with a higher prevalence (25%) in African-American patients. [27].

The majority of cases of sarcoidosis uveitis are bilateral, and around *90%* are chronic[21] The prevalence of the different subtypes of uveitis varies from study to study, due to the terminology used. In one study, of 112 eyes with sarcoidosis uveitis, 28% had anterior uveitis, 38% intermediate uveitis, 12% posterior uveitis and 22% panuveitis. [21] Another study reported a prevalence of 46% for intermediate uveitis, 15% for anterior uveitis and 38% for panuveitis. A Japanese study found 75% iritis and 67% retinal vasculitis. [16].

The prevalence of sarcoidosis in patients with multifocal chorioretinitis varies according to diagnostic criteria and the extent of investigations carried out in different studies. One study showed a prevalence of biopsy-proven and presumptive sarcoidosis of 68% in 37 patients with multifocal chorioretinitis, [29]. Another study reported a rate of 39%[30]. It should be noted that the first study included a chest CT scan in 62% of patients,[29] while only 26% of patients in the second study received one. [30] The ACCESS study (Case Control Etiologic Study of Sarcoidosis) demonstrated that allelic variations in the HLA-DRB1 locus are a significant contributing factor to sarcoidosis. The HLADRB1*0401 allele was associated with ocular involvement in both African-American and Caucasian populations, with an odds ratio of 3.49. [31]

Phenotypes of patients with sarcoidosis uveitis :

Two phenotypes are classically described: the first involves young subjects aged 20 to 30 of varied ethnic origin, with more often than not acute uveitis associated with extraophthalmological manifestations. The second involves mainly women over 50 of European origin, more often with isolated chronic uveitis [32,33].

A third group of patients has recently been identified, corresponding to patients of European origin who are older than the first group; here, the proportion of acute and chronic uveitis is equivalent, and the visual prognosis is better than in the classic group of young patients [34]. However, these studies were carried out in European countries and should be interpreted with caution for other populations.

Using cluster analysis, Schupp et al. showed an association between ocular, cardiac, cutaneous and central nervous system manifestations [35]. Furthermore, Van Swol et al. recently reported that 16% of patients with ocular sarcoidosis showed signs of cardiac sarcoidosis on electrocardiogram at the time of diagnosis of ocular sarcoidosis [36]. In contrast, in our center, we showed that out of 294 patients with sarcoidosis uveitis, only 2.4% developed cardiac involvement [37]. Niederer et al. also reported 4.4% cardiac sarcoids in their retrospective cohort of sarcoidosis uveitis [38]. However, particular attention should be paid to patients with previously diagnosed sarcoidosis or those who develop systemic sarcoidosis during follow-up.

3. Clinical manifestations of ocular sarcoidosis

The initial symptoms of sarcoidosis may be eye problems, leading to severe visual impairment. The condition is characterized by granulomatous inflammation that can affect various parts of the eye and its associated tissues.

- Uveitis and fundus abnormalities

Uveitis is an inflammation of the eye that primarily affects uveal tissues such as the iris, ciliary body and choroid, as well as the entire intraocular structure. As described by the Working Group on Standardization of Uveitis Nomenclature, a distinction is generally made between four types of uveitis, depending on the primary location of inflammation: anterior uveitis, which affects the iris and ciliary body; intermediate uveitis, which affects the vitreous body and retinal periphery; posterior uveitis, which affects the retina and choroid; and panuveitis, which involves all intraocular tissues. Sarcoidosis can cause all these forms of uveitis: anterior, intermediate, posterior or panuveitis.

Uveitis is also classified according to etiology: infectious uveitis (16% of all uveitis), non-infectious uveitis (47%) and unclassified uveitis (37%) [39]. In infectious uveitis, intraocular inflammation is caused by infectious pathogens such as viruses, bacteria, fungi and parasites. In non-infectious uveitis - such as sarcoidosis, VKH disease, Behcet's disease, sympathetic ophthalmia, uveitis associated with inflammatory bowel disease, uveitis associated with juvenile idiopathic arthritis, tubulointerstitial nephritis, uveitis associated with uveitis syndrome and HLA-B27-associated anterior uveitis. The precise pathogenesis of the latter is not fully elucidated, but immunological and autoimmune mechanisms are thought to play an important role.

Uveitis can present in different anatomical types in the context of sarcoidosis: anterior, intermediate, posterior or panuveitis [40].

Anterior uveitis is the most common form, accounting for 41% to 81% of cases of sarcoidosis uveitis [41,42]. In specialized centers treating the most severe forms, panuveitis is the most common presentation [43,44,45]. It is characterized by bilateral, granulomatous involvement with a symmetrical course in both eyes, although it may remain unilateral in 25% of cases [5,46]. In 2021, the SUN working group published classification criteria for sarcoidosis uveitis, while the IWOS group proposed seven suggestive ophthalmological signs and specific classification criteria [47,48]. The American Thoracic Society's 2020 recommendations suggest a systematic ophthalmological examination in any patient with sarcoidosis, even in the absence of ocular symptoms, although the level of evidence remains low and a recent study identified no benefit for screening asymptomatic patients [49,50].

3.1. anterior uveitis:

Anterior uveitis is the most common sign of sarcoidosis uveitis. It is characterized by inflammation of the anterior chamber of the eye in the form of iritis, iridocyclitis or anterior hyalitis [51]. Symptoms may include redness, blurred vision, ocular pain and sensitivity to light.

It may present acutely, with a sudden onset and duration of less than three months, but is often chronic, with relapses occurring less than three months after treatment has been discontinued [51].An increase in intraocular pressure may be observed, either due to the ocular inflammation itself, or as a result of treatment [47,52]. Anterior synechiae (between cornea and iris) and posterior synechiae (between iris and lens) are typically present [47]. Sarcoidosis uveitis is often granulomatous, manifesting as large retrocorneal precipitates or iris nodules located near the pupil (Koeppe nodules) or in the iris stroma (Busacca nodules) (Figure I)or in the trabecular meshwork.(figure) Iris nodules are usually associated with more severe inflammation. Without appropriate treatment, severe anterior uveitis can lead to complications such as anterior segment deformities and cataract formation.

However, granulomatous uveitis is not specific to sarcoidosis, as other pathologies such as tuberculosis can also present with granulomatous uveitis. Moreover, in some studies, more than half of patients have non-granulomatous uveitis, particularly in cases of Lofgren's syndrome [4,47,53].

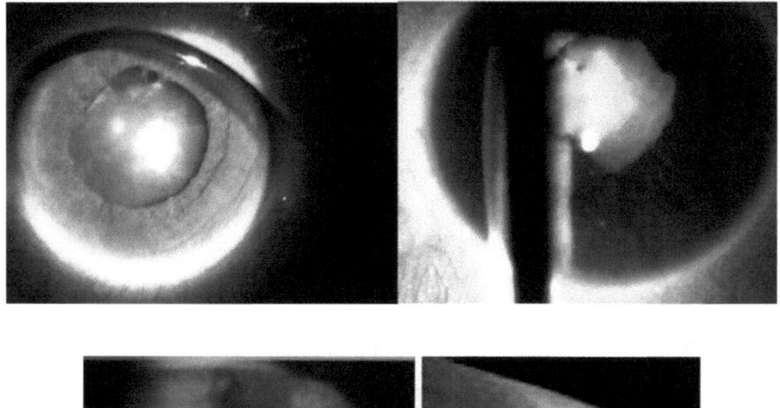
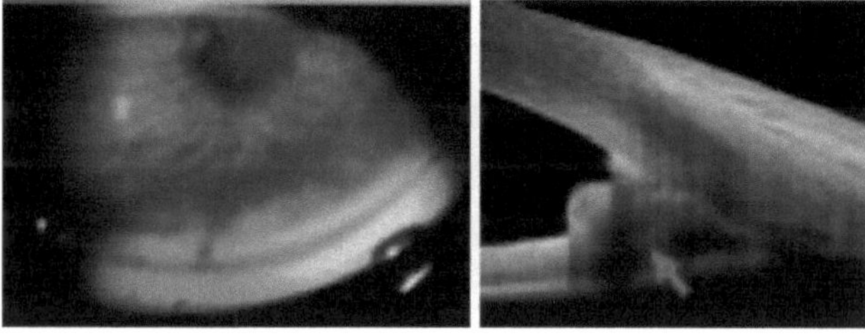

Figure: A: SA photo showing an iris and ciliary body granuloma in a patient with suspected sarcoidosis

8: OCT SA showing a hyporeflective iris prominence process

3.2. Intermediate uveitis

In intermediate uveitis, inflammation is mainly localized in the vitreous humor, presenting as pars planitis, posterior cyclitis or hyalitis [51,54]. Intermediate uveitis is most often idiopathic, but sarcoidosis accounts for 7-18% of cases, making it a frequent etiology alongside multiple sclerosis [55,56,57]. Intermediate uveitis is also common in ocular sarcoidosis. Patients may present with floating bodies and blurred vision.

The most common features of intermediate uveitis in sarcoidosis are the presence of "ant-egg" vitreous opacities that may be organized into "pearly exudates". The main causes of vision loss in patients with intermediate uveitis are cystoid macular edema, followed by vitreous opacity, epiretinal membrane opacity, optic neuritis and glaucoma [56].

3.3. Posterior uveitis

Posterior uveitis involves inflammation of the retina and/or choroid [40]. Fundus examination is a key component of the clinical examination, but the use of complementary examinations such as optical coherence tomography (OCT) and angiography is very useful. Posterior uveitis accounts for 5-28% of ocular sarcoidosis cases [4,5,42,46,58]. Although less frequent than anterior involvement, it poses a greater threat to the patient's vision [59]. Authentic choroidal granulomas in the peripheral retina or around the optic nerve have been described, but multifocal choroiditis (Figure 2) is much more common [47,60,61]. Both lesions can progress to atrophic scarring of the pigment epithelium. Retinal and preretinal nodules have rarely been reported as the only posterior manifestations of ocular sarcoidosis without choroidal involvement [62].

In severe forms, these granulomas can lead to exudative retinal detachment [63]. Although they may be present in other types of uveitis, the presence of granuloma has a higher predictive value in ocular sarcoidosis than in other forms of granulomatous uveitis. [65].

OCT/angiography can be useful for visualizing changes in granuloma formation and assessing microvascular and perfusion alterations [64,65]. Indeed, retinal vasculitis is often associated with sarcoidosis. Ten to seventeen percent of patients suffer from segmental periphlebitis [47].

The classic perivascular infiltrates and sheaths, known as candle spots, are rare and can sometimes only be identified by fluorescein angiography [67]. This condition is classically observed in the acute phase of uveitis and is generally associated with a poorer visual prognosis and more frequent relapses [68]. Some vasculitides are associated with vascular occlusions (mainly venous), which may be complicated by retinal neovascularization in *5%* of cases (in association with ischemia and chronic inflammation) [69].

Ocular sarcoidosis can also present multiple inflammatory macroaneurysms. Bilaterality is also an important feature of ocular sarcoidosis. Arterial involvement in sarcoidosis is rare [70]. Cystoid macular edema is observed in 19-72% of cases of posterior uveitis. It is important to remember that sarcoidosis affecting the posterior segment may be accompanied by central nervous system involvement in 25-30% of patients [71].

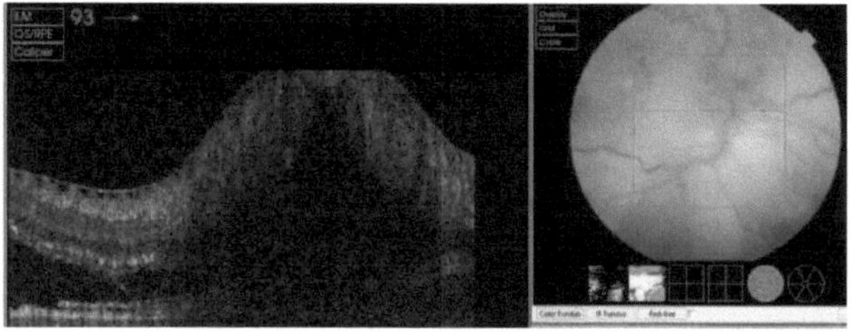

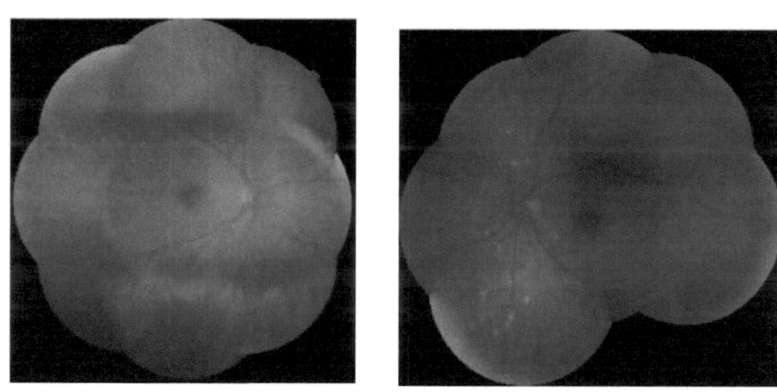

Figure 2. bilateral multifocal choroiditis

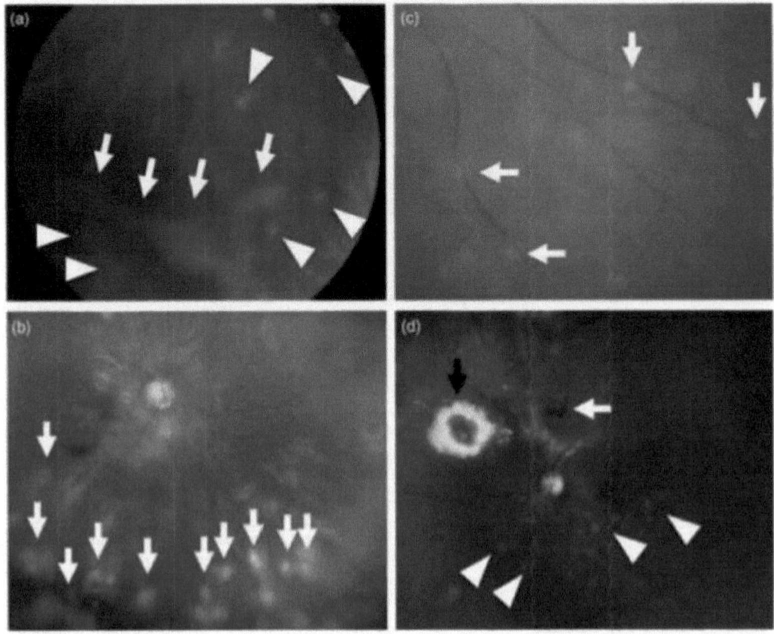

Figure: posterior segment damage in srcoidosis (a) vitreous opacities in the form of pearly exudates (arrows) and multiple chorioretinal lesions (arrowheads) (b) multiple fresh chorioretinal lesions (arrows) (c) periphlebitis (arrows) (d) multiple arrows macroaneurysms surrounded by hard white exudates (arrows) and multiple chorioretinal lesions (arrowheads), by takasi et al [65].

3.4. Panuveitis

Panuveitis affects all structures of the eye, and includes all the lesions we have already described [40]. They are the most frequent form of uveitis in tertiary centers, and are estimated to account for 37% of sarcoidosis uveitis by the SUN working group [5,47]. Sarcoidosis is the systemic disease most frequently associated with panuveitis, ahead of tuberculosis and Behçet's disease [55,72,73].

3.5. Ocular complications

Even anterior uveitis can lead to ocular complications, including band keratopathy, cataracts and glaucoma. These complications are both secondary to the inflammatory process and iatrogenic on corticosteroids [32]. More seriously, cystoid macular edema (Figure 3) is the main cause of vision loss in sarcoid uveitis [43]. Epiretinal membranes may develop in severe vitreoretinal inflammation and may be responsible for retinal traction, leading to retinal tears and rhegmatogenous retinal detachment [74].

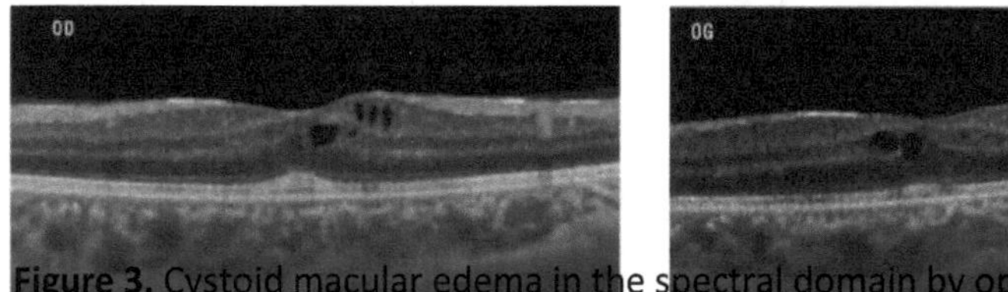

Figure 3. Cystoid macular edema in the spectral domain by optical coherence tomography.

Examples of clinical manifestations of ocular sarcoidosis

Eye structures	Ophthalmic manifestations
- Eyelids	Eyelid granuloma, madarosis (loss of eyelashes), poliosis (whitening of eyelashes), entropion, trichiasis, lagoghthalmos (if associated with facial paralysis).
- Conjunctive	Conjunctival nodules or granulomas, conjunctivitis, symblepharon, conjunctival scarring
- Episclerotic/sclerotic	Episcleritis, scleritis
- Cornea	Peripheral ulcerative keratitis, interstitial keratitis, exposure keratopathy, band keratopathy
- Trabecular meshwork and anterior chamber angle	Trabecular granuloma, peripheral anterior synechiae, ocular hypertension, glaucoma
-Iris	Anterior uveitis (iritis), iris nodules/granulomas, posterior synechiae, pupillary anomalies
- Lens	Cataracts
- Pars plana/vitreous	Intermediate uveitis
- Retina	Retinitis, retinal vasculitis, macular edema
- Choroid	Choroiditis, granuloma
- Optic nerve	Papillitis, papilledema (increased intracranial pressure due to neurosarcoid), granuloma, optic neuropathy (compressive or infiltrative), optic atrophy
- Tear gland	Granuloma, dacryoadenitis, keratoconjunctivitis sicca (dry eye)
- Nasolacrimal drainage system	Nasolacrimal duct obstruction
- Extraocular muscles and other orbital tissues	Granuloma, strabismus, proptosis, optic nerve compression
- Intracranial lesions involving the visual pathways	Diminished vision, visual field defects, abnormal pupillary response, abnormal eye movements

3.5.1. Optic nerve damage and neuro-ophthalmic manifestations

Neurosarcoidosis is often referred to as "simulative" because of its polymorphism of symptoms, which can lead to confusion with several pathologies. Symptoms vary according to the location of granulomas and associated inflammatory complications. They may include decreased vision or visual field defects due to damage to the optic nerve and its visual pathway, edema of the optic nerve head due to increased intracranial pressure, abnormal eye movements, pupillary abnormalities, visual hallucinations, encephalopathy, vasculopathy, peripheral neuropathy, myopathy, seizures, aseptic meningitis, hydrocephalus, spinal cord involvement and psychiatric symptoms. [75]. Cranial neuropathy is the most common manifestation of neurosarcoidosis, mainly affecting the optic and facial nerves. [76]. Optic nerve involvement may present as granulomas or nodules, papilledema or optic atrophy.

Papilledema may be associated with severe posterior uveitis, periphlebitis or direct granuloma involvement of the nerve or its sheath. [77]. Irreversible impairment of visual acuity is observed in more than half of patients with direct optic nerve damage. Facial paresis is also common, and may result from inflammation of the parotid gland, a meningeal reaction or direct compression. [78]. This paresis can cause eyelid closure problems, leading to ocular complications such as exposure keratitis, epiphora and ectropion. Severe corneal ulcers can lead to permanent vision loss.

It's important to note that these ocular and neurological manifestations may vary from one individual to another, and that other symptoms may also be present.

In neurosarcoidosis, acquired abnormal eye movements, such as nystagmus, may be observed, as well as pupillary anomalies and visual hallucinations. These ocular symptoms may be due to the direct effect of granulomas or inflammatory sequelae on nerves and associated structures. [79]. It should be noted that ocular manifestations may vary from individual to individual and are not always present in all patients with neurosarcoidosis. [80].

3.5.2. Diseases of the eyelids and ocular surface

Dermatological manifestations of sarcoidosis are well documented. Partial or total eyelid involvement may be observed, with periorbital erythematous swelling possibly the only sign of ocular sarcoidosis. [81,82]. Erythematous lesions of the eyelid may vary in size; small papules[83], nodules(figure), large masses which may mimic palpebral tumours or skin scars[84]. Cases have been reported where chronic eyelid nodules have led to eyelid deformities, mucocutaneous notches, entropion, trichiasis and extensive eyelid destruction.

Conjunctival involvement is also frequent, with conjunctival nodules observed mainly in the palpebral conjunctiva. Cases of acute follicular conjunctivitis, chronic cicatricial conjunctivitis with symblépharon and large conjunctival granulomas have been reported. [85,86].

Scleritis, although rarely associated with sarcoidosis, can present in different forms, including diffuse anterior, nodular anterior or posterior scleritis. [87,88]. Sarcoidosis-associated scleritis is generally non-necrotizing and responds well to oral corticosteroids. However, it should be noted that sarcoidosis is not the most common cause of necrotizing scleritis. [90].

Ocular sarcoidosis can also affect the cornea. Superficial punctate keratitis is the most common corneal manifestation, often associated with keratoconjunctivitis sicca. Calcium deposits on Bowman's subepithelial layer can cause peripheral banded opacities, also known as banded keratopathy. [91]. Interstitial keratitis, characterized by corneal inflammation with signs of posterior uveitis and optic disc edema, has also been reported. In some cases, severe peripheral ulcerative keratitis with corneal perforation may occur. [92].

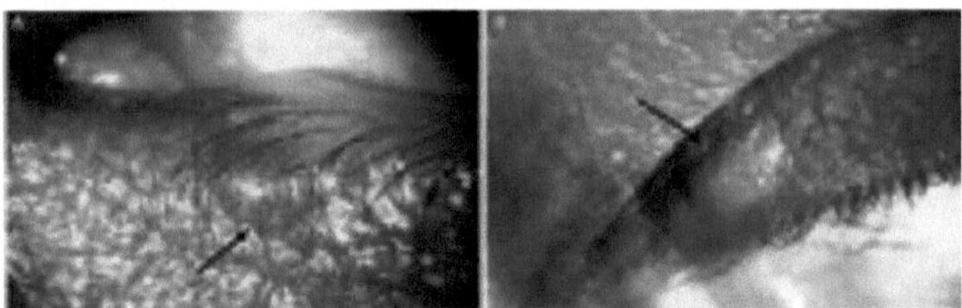

Figure: Sarcoidosis palpebral nodules in a 47-year-old patient whose biopsy reveals granulomatous infallamtion without caseous necrosis, confirming the diagnosis of sarcoidosis.

3.5.3. The lacrimal system and keratoconjunctivitis sicca (KCS)

In orbital sarcoidosis, the lacrimal gland is frequently affected. Histopathological studies have shown that the lacrimal gland is the main orbital organ affected in 42% to 63% of biopsy-confirmed cases of sarcoidosis. [93,94] Infiltration of the lacrimal gland has been observed in 30% of sarcoidosis cases. It is often bilateral and may be associated with parotid swelling and dacryoadenitis (Heerfordt syndrome). [93]

Patients with lacrimal gland involvement may present with variable symptoms. [95] Marked hypertrophy of the gland may result in a palpable mass, mechanical ptosis, eyelid deformity or other compression-related symptoms. Typical features seen on CT scan are diffuse lacrimal gland hypertrophy with homogeneous enhancement.

Dry eye syndrome is a frequent consequence of inflammation and infiltration of the lacrimal gland in sarcoidosis, leading to reduced production of aqueous tears. Studies have focused mainly on the main lacrimal gland, but there is no specific mention of involvement of the accessory lacrimal glands.

The main lacrimal glands located in the anterolateral part of the orbit are responsible for the secretion of reflex tears, while the small accessory lacrimal glands located in the eyelid and conjunctiva produce the majority of basal tears. Both the main and accessory lacrimal glands may be affected in people with severe sarcoidosis-related dry eyes. Dry eyes can cause symptoms such as irritation, tearing, corneal problems such as epitheliopathy, abrasion, infection and permanent scarring.

The lacrimal drainage system, comprising the lacrimal points, canaliculi, lacrimal sac and nasolacrimal duct, can be directly affected by granulomatous inflammation due to sarcoidosis, resulting in lacrimal obstruction and excessive lacrimation (epiphora)[96,97];

3.5.4. Damage to the orbit

In addition to the lacrimal gland, sarcoidosis can also affect other structures in the orbit, such as orbital fat, extraocular muscles and the optic nerve sheath. [93]

Histopathological studies revealed that the main symptoms in patients with orbital sarcoidosis requiring biopsy were a palpable mass and eyelid swelling. [93,94] Other symptoms include displacement of the eyeball, proptosis (exophthalmos), redness, pain, decreased vision, lacrimation and diplopia. In 34-50% of cases of biopsy-confirmed orbital sarcoidosis, concomitant systemic sarcoidosis has been observed. [93,94]

Orbital lesions were well-demarcated in 85-90% of cases, while 10-15% were diffuse or infiltrative. These lesions are generally solid, although rarely cystic. [94]; They are mainly located in the anterior orbit, particularly in the anteroinferior region. [98];The presence of an orbital mass due to sarcoidosis can lead to occlusion of the central retinal artery, resulting in permanent blindness. [99].

3.5.5. Glaucoma and cataracts

In patients with sarcoid uveitis, elevated intraocular pressure (IOP) and the development of glaucoma are common. Studies have shown that sarcoid uveitis associated with glaucoma can lead to severe visual loss in some patients. [100]; Ocular hypertension and glaucoma may be due to trabecular meshwork dysfunction caused by edema or obstruction by inflammatory cells. Severe or chronic inflammation in the anterior chamber of the eye can lead to angle-closure glaucoma due to the formation of peripheral anterior synechiae. A Japanese study revealed a high incidence of abnormal findings on gonioscopic examination in patients with systemic sarcoidosis, such as trabecular nodules and tent-like peripheral anterior synechiae.

Patients with uveitic glaucoma have an increased risk of failure during filtering surgery. [101]; In addition, IOP elevation may be due to mass effects in the orbit or to side effects of corticosteroid therapy.

Cataract formation is also common in patients with sarcoidosis uveitis, which causes visual impairment. All forms of corticosteroid therapy, whether topical, regional or systemic, can contribute to cataract development and elevated intraocular pressure.

4. Diagnostic approach

4.1. Sarcoidosis: a difficult diagnosis

Sarcoidosis is a disease that can affect different ocular tissues simultaneously, manifesting itself in different ways. Patients may present with acute anterior uveitis with lacrimal gland enlargement, bilateral multifocal choroiditis with conjunctival nodules, or peripheral ulcerative keratitis with orbital inflammation. It is important to consider sarcoidosis as one of the differential diagnoses in patients with multiple ocular tissue involvement.

Tissue biopsy is considered the gold standard for the diagnosis of sarcoidosis. Biopsy samples are usually taken from the lungs, lymph nodes, skin, conjunctiva, lacrimal glands or orbital tissues. However, it can sometimes be difficult to access suspicious lesions, and biopsy may not be desirable from the patient's point of view. The lungs and hilar lymph nodes are the organs most frequently affected. Imaging tests such as chest X-ray, thoracic CT scan and sometimes gallium scintigraphy can contribute to the diagnosis. Some patients with sarcoidosis may have elevated serum levels of calcium, angiotensin-converting enzyme (ACE) and/or lysozymes.

Sarcoidosis uveitis has no specific clinical features, and it is important to exclude other serious conditions such as lymphoma when diagnosing uveitis [74,75]. Granulomatous uveitis is also associated with other diseases such as tuberculosis, syphilis, Vogt-Koyanagi-Harada syndrome, toxoplasmosis and herpetic uveitis [76]. Choroidal granulomas are frequently seen in tuberculosis, making differential diagnosis difficult [77,78].

There is no specific marker for easy diagnosis of sarcoidosis, and systemic investigations are necessary. The diagnosis of sarcoidosis is based on histological evidence of epithelioid giant cell granulomas without caseous necrosis, but intraocular biopsies carry risks for vision, and blind conjunctival biopsies remain controversial [79,80-82]. In practice, the diagnosis of sarcoidosis uveitis is often made on the basis of a combination of clinical and paraclinical data. International criteria from the International Workshop on Ocular Sarcoidosis (IWOS) have been proposed for the diagnosis of ocular sarcoidosis, and a revised classification was presented in 2019 [48].

For all cases of uveitis, a minimal workup should be performed, including a complete blood count, C-reactive protein measurement, syphilis serology, tuberculin skin tests (or IFN-y release assays, IGRA) and chest imaging. A positive tuberculin test or a positive IGRA is an exclusion criterion in the SUN classification [50]. However, in France, where tuberculosis is not very endemic, 12% of patients with sarcoidosis uveitis meeting the inclusion criteria had a positive IGRA [85]. In case of doubt, empirical antituberculosis treatment may be considered [86].

According to these experts, the diagnosis of ocular sarcoidosis is based on a 4-step approach: [48].

1. **Eliminate all other causes of granulomatous uveitis.**

2. **Look for clinical signs compatible with ocular sarcoidosis (OS):**

   1 granulomatous retrodescemetic precipitates and/or iris nodules (Koeppe or Busacca)
   2 nodules in the iridocorneal angle and/or anterior synechiae;
   3 snowballs vitréens;
   4 multiple peripheral chorioretinal lesions (active or atrophic);
   5 segmental and/or nodular periphlebitis (or "candle-spot" appearance) and/or macroaneurysm in an inflamed eye;
   6 nodule(s) or granuloma(s) of the papilla;

3. **Analyze the results of complementary examinations compatible with sarcoidosis**

   ocular: (Part of the work-up for suspected ocular sarcoidosis)

   1- negative tuberculin TST;
   2- Bilateral hilar adenopathy on chest X-ray and/or CT scan;
   3- 3-Elevation of angiotensin-converting enzyme.
   4- -Elevated serum lysozyme.
   5- -High CD4/CD8 ratio (>3.5) in bronchoalveolar lavage fluid.

6- Abnormal accumulation of gallium-67 on scintigraphy or 18F-fluorodeoxyglucose on positron emission tomography.

7- Lymphopenia.

8- Parenchymal lung changes compatible with sarcoidosis, determined by pulmonologists or radiologists.

4. <u>**Propose a conclusion on the possibility of ocular sarcoidosis :**</u>

Group 1: Diagnosis certain = confirmed

Positive biopsy (in practice, eye biopsies are never carried out due to the iatrogenic risks associated with sampling...). A conjunctival biopsy is cost-effective in cases of associated follicular conjunctivitis; biopsy of a palpable adenopathy, lacrimal gland or lung parenchyma during bronchial fibroscopy in the event of an orienting sign.

Group 2: presumptive diagnosis in the absence of an ocular biopsy, but when thoracic imaging reveals bilateral hilar adenopathies associated with two compatible intraocular signs.

Group 3: Probable diagnosis in the absence of bilateral hilar adenopathies, but when three ocular signs are present and associated with two other positive complementary tests.

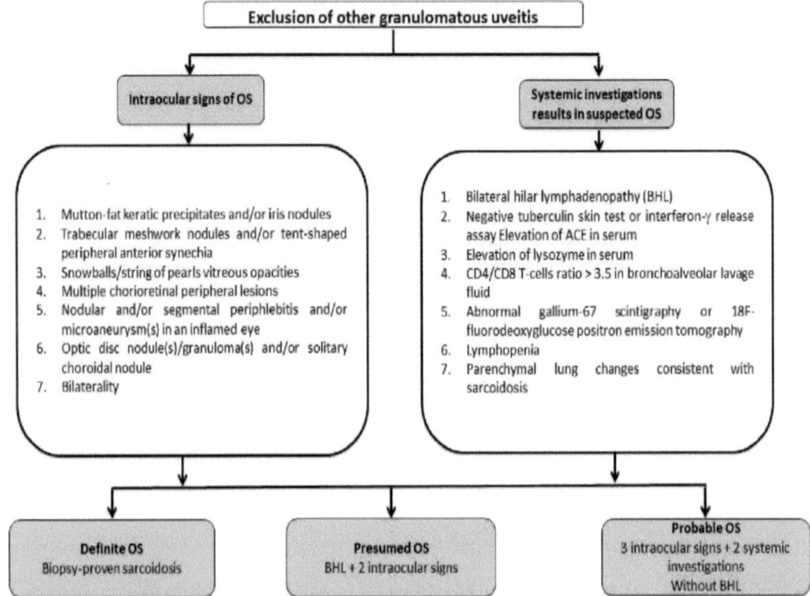

Figure. Revised diagnostic criteria for ocular sarcoldosis (OS) as recommended by the International

Workshop on Ocular Sarcoidosis (IWOS)", [48,71].

Abbreviations: BHL: bilateral hilar lymphadenopathy; ACE: angiotensin-converting enzyme; OS: ocular sarcoidosis.

Table Classification criteria for sarcoidosis uveitis recommended by the Standardization of Uveitis Nomenclature (SUN), taken from Standardization of Uveitis Nomenclature (SUN) Working.

Group classification criteria for sarcoidosis-associated uveitis. *Am. J. Ophthalmol.* **2021** [47], with permission from Elsevier.

__Criteria__
1.   Uveitic image compatible, either:
a.   Anterior uveitis or
b.   Intermediate or anterior/intermediate uveitis or
c.   Posterior uveitis with choroiditis (paucifocal choroidal nodule(s) or multifocal choroiditis) or
d.   Panuveitis with choroiditis or retinal vascular sheath or retinal vascular occlusion.
ET
2.   Evidence of sarcoidosis, i.e. :
a.   Tissue biopsy demonstrating non-caseous granulomas or
b.   Bilateral hilar adenopathy on thoracic imaging.

__Exclusions__
1. Positive serology for syphilis using a treponemal test.
2. Evidence of infection with *Mycobacterium tuberculosis*[*,1,2] , i.e. :
a. Histologically or microbiologically confirmed *M. tuberculosis* infection[b] or
b. Positive interferon-y release assay (IGRA)[3] or
c. Positive tuberculin skin test[d]

4.2. In search of serum biomarkers predictive of sarcoidosis

No biomarker currently available is sufficiently reliable to make the diagnosis of sarcoidosis. Anti-retin antibodies have been identified in ocular sarcoidosis and other types of uveitis, but their sensitivity and specificity are not yet sufficient to be recommended. Lymphopenia, a decrease in the number of lymphocytes in the blood, is a criterion included in the diagnostic criteria for sarcoidosis [48], but its sensitivity and specificity vary from study to study. Angiotensin-converting enzyme (ACE) is one of the best-known and most widely used markers, but its sensitivity and specificity also vary in different series of studies. [113]. Serum lysozyme assay is another marker studied, but its interpretation alone must be cautious due to its possible increase in other conditions. Other markers such as soluble interleukin-2 receptor (sIL-2R), chitotriosidase and Krebs von den Lungen (KL-6) are also being studied, but their clinical use is not yet established. [114,115]. In practice, the combination of serum biomarkers with morphological examinations is often necessary to improve the diagnosis of sarcoidosis. [85,116].

4.3. Imaging modalities

Chest CT is probably the most frequently used imaging test for the detection of sarcoidosis today, supplanting chest X-ray [117]. Parenchymal lung abnormalities compatible with sarcoidosis are now included in the IWOS criteria for ocular sarcoidosis, provided that the imaging is reviewed by pulmonologists or specialist radiologists [48]. More recently, nuclear imaging with 18F-fluorodeoxyglucose positron emission tomography (18F-FDG PET) has become an imaging modality of choice for the diagnosis and management of sarcoidosis, although large-scale prospective studies are needed to clarify its place in the diagnostic workup [118]. 18F-FDG PET would be of interest: (1) in cases of suspected extra-pulmonary involvement, such as neurosarcoidosis or cardiac sarcoidosis, where it may help define a target for biopsy, (2) in pulmonary fibrosis to assess active lesions that may regress with anti-inflammatory treatment, (3) in cardiac sarcoidosis to assess response to treatment (cardiac 18F-FDG-PET), (4) in the most complex cases to assess therapeutic response and risk of relapse [119]. Advanced age at diagnosis, the presence of posterior synechiae and increased CEA levels were significantly associated with abnormal 18F-FDG PET [120,121]. In this study, although the chest CT was normal, 30% of patients with suspected sarcoidosis uveitis had hypermetabolic foci on 18F-FDG PET [121].

However, we must remain cautious about the contribution of 18F-FDG PET compared with chest CT, particularly in the differential diagnosis with ocular tuberculosis, where 18F-FDG PET is not a diagnostic tool.Contradictory data exist in regions where tuberculosis is endemic [122].

4.4 Invasive investigations

Bronchoalveolar lavage (BAL) has been studied for the diagnosis of sarcoidosis uveitis.

It has a sensitivity of 63% and specificity of 75% in patients with histologically proven sarcoidosis [123]. Lymphocytic alveolitis with a predominance of CD4 T lymphocytes (CD4/CD8 ratio > 3.5) may be observed, even in the absence of radiological abnormalities. However, the biopsy is usually not positive when the chest CT is normal. [99,124].

Other studies have explored CD4/CD8 ratios in other biological fluids such as vitreous fluid, showing significantly higher levels in patients with sarcoidosis compared with other causes of uveitis. [124].

Work is in progress to identify cytokine profiles in the aqueous humor in order to distinguish sarcoidosis from tuberculosis. [125]. Proteomic analysis of vitreous humor samples is also being carried out to search for new biomarkers. [126,127]. However, the invasive nature of these samples limits their widespread use. [128].

Minor salivary gland biopsy (MSGB) shows poor diagnostic performance in ocular sarcoidosis, with a sensitivity of 5.2% and 3% in studies.

[129,130]. Furthermore, MSGB cannot exclude tuberculosis, which is an important part of the differential diagnosis of granulomas on MSGB. Therefore, MSGB should only be considered in patients with elevated serum ACE or compatible CT abnormalities. [130].

Transbronchial lymph node aspiration guided by endobronchial ultrasonography performs well in the diagnosis of sarcoidosis in general [131], but there are few data specific to ocular sarcoidosis. [132].

5.5. Algorithm for evaluating patients with suspected sarcoidosis uveitis

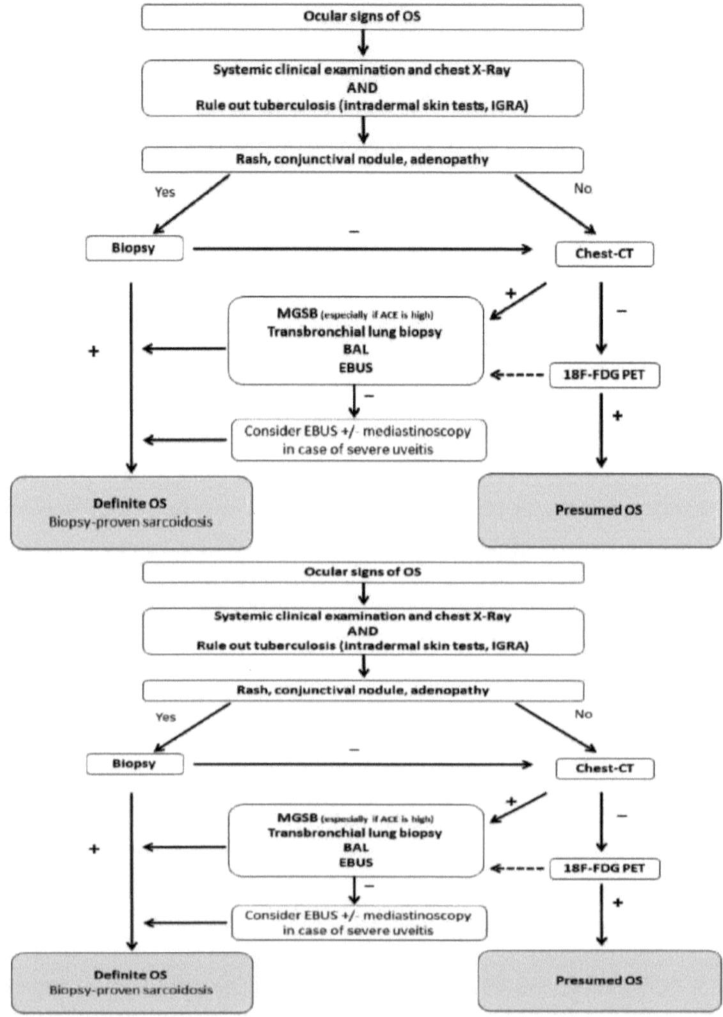

Figure Diagnostic algorithm for suspected ocular sarcoidosis [71,102,133].
Abbreviations: ACE: angiotensin-converting enzyme; BAL: bronchoalveolar lavage; EBUS: endoscopic ultrasound-guided fine-needle aspiration of intrathoracic lymph nodes; IGRA: interferon-y release assay; MSGB: minor salivary gland biopsy; OS: ocular sarcoidosis; 18F-FDG PET: 18-fluorodeoxyglucose positron emission tomography.

5. Visual prognosis of sarcoidosis uveitis

The visual prognosis of ocular sarcoid uveitis is generally good [134]. Less than 10% of patients experience severe visual impairment, defined as visual acuity below 20/200 [43,44,135,136]. Complications of ocular inflammation are very common, in particular cataracts, which affect up to 73% of patients depending on the study [134,137]. In the report by Suzuki et al, cataract was present in 62.2% of cases, glaucoma in 28.5%, epiretinal membrane in 24.1% and cystoid macular edema in 22.6% [134]. Nevertheless, the main cause of vision loss remains cystoid macular edema (a consequence of uveitis) [43]. Several risk factors have been associated with a poor functional prognosis, such as late age of onset, African-American origin, female gender, underlying chronic systemic sarcoidosis, posterior segment involvement, chronic cystoid macular edema, multifocal choroiditis, persistent ocular inflammation and glaucoma [4,44,134,138]. In a French tertiary center, just over a quarter of patients recovered from their disease; two variables were associated with this favorable outcome: Caucasian origin and previous localization of uveitis [129]. For women of childbearing age, the evolution during pregnancy seems reassuring, although few data exist. Our recent retrospective work suggests that it evolves in the same way as other uveitis (i.e., with a decrease in the frequency of attacks during the last trimester) [140].

6. Treatments

The visual prognosis of ocular sarcoid uveitis is generally favorable, with less than 10% of patients presenting with severe visual impairment. Ocular complications are common, particularly cataracts, which affect up to 73% of patients. Cystoid macular edema is the main cause of vision loss. Certain risk factors are associated with a poor functional prognosis, such as late age of onset, African-American origin, female gender, underlying chronic systemic sarcoidosis, posterior segment involvement, chronic cystoid macular edema, multifocal choroiditis, persistent ocular inflammation and glaucoma. A significant proportion of patients can recover from the disease, particularly those of Caucasian origin and with a previous localization of uveitis. For women of childbearing age, the course during pregnancy appears generally favorable.

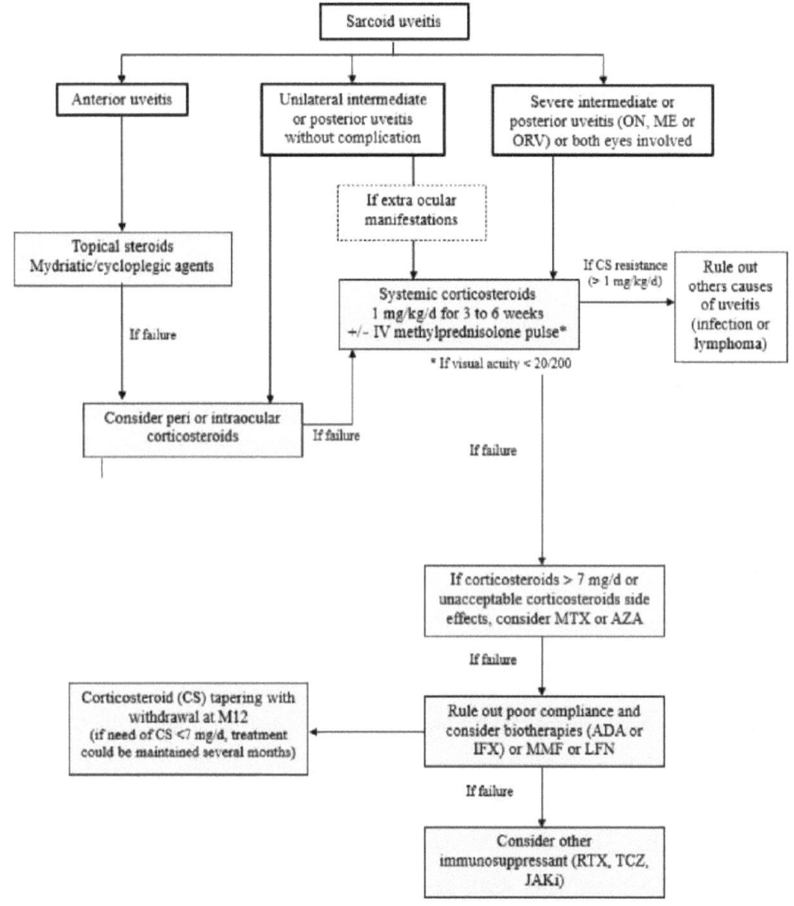

Figure. Therapeutic management of ocular sarcoidosis, after [133].
Abbreviations: ON: optic neuritis; ME: macular edema; ORV: occlusive retinal vasculitis; MTX: methotrexate; AZA: azathioprine; MMF: mycophenolate mofetil; LFN: leflunomide; RTX: rituximab; TCZ: tocilizumab; JAKi: Janus kinase inhibitor; IV: intravenous.

The main objectives of ocular sarcoidosis management are to restore vision and prevent complications associated with inflammation. Corticosteroid therapy, whether topical, regional or systemic, is the mainstay of treatment. Other immunomodulators may be required in certain patients who are dependent on, unresponsive to or intolerant of corticosteroid therapy.

7. Treatment of sarcoidosis uveitis

7.1. Topical corticosteroids, such as prednisolone acetate and difluprednate, are commonly used to treat anterior uveitis. Dosage can be adjusted according to the degree of inflammation, ranging from once a day to once an hour. Difluprednate is a more potent drug and may be as effective as prednisolone acetate in treating anterior uveitis. [14û]; However, these drugs can have undesirable side effects, such as increased intraocular pressure and cataract progression.

Topical corticosteroids are mainly used to treat inflammation of the anterior chamber of the eye, but may not be sufficient to control inflammation of the posterior segment. However, they may be effective in treating cystoid macular edema associated with severe anterior uveitis.

7.2. Cycloplegic eye drops are used to relieve pain caused by ciliary spasm and to prevent or rupture posterior synechiae, which are common in patients with moderate to severe anterior chamber inflammation. Short-acting drugs, such as cyclopentolate, are generally used in acute cases, while longer-acting agents, such as atropine, may be administered in cases of chronic or severe anterior chamber inflammation.

7.3. Regional corticosteroid injections and implants are treatment options for uveitis with posterior segment involvement, or when the response to topical corticosteroids is inadequate. Depot injections can be performed periocularly (around the eye) or intravitreally (in the vitreous of the eye). Periocular injections can be administered transcutaneously (through the skin) or transconjunctivally (through the conjunctiva). According to current practice, injection into the orbital floor is generally performed through the skin of the inferolateral eyelid. Triamcinolone acetonide, at a dose of 20 to 40 mg, is the most widely used drug. Other alternatives include betamethasone and methylprednisolone, both of which have a shorter duration of action than triamcinolone acetonide. Injections can be repeated 4 to 6 weeks after the initial treatment.

Intravitreal injections of triamcinolone acetonide, usually 1 to 4 mg, can be given when periocular injections fail to control inflammation. The effects of these injections may last from 3 to 6 months after each administration. It is important to monitor patients carefully for any rise in intraocular pressure (IOP). The procedure can be performed clinically under topical or subconjunctival anesthesia.

A biodegradable intraocular implant containing 700 micrograms of dexamethasone, administered through the pars plana using a 22-gauge applicator, has been approved for the treatment of uveitis involving the posterior segment of the eye. A study of its efficacy and safety in persistent cystoid macular edema associated with uveitis showed that a single dexamethasone implant was effective in improving vision and reducing macular edema in the majority of patients. However, around 65% of patients experienced a recurrence of cystoid macular edema after 6 months. [142] A study comparing intravitreal triamcinolone injections with dexamethasone implants in cystoid macular edema secondary to retinal vein occlusion showed similar results and a similar incidence of side effects. [143].

A sustained-release fluocinolone acetonide implant has been approved in the USA for the treatment of chronic non-infectious posterior uveitis. This implant is surgically inserted into the vitreous cavity and can release the drug for an average period of 30 months. It is effective in controlling inflammation in the majority of implanted eyes. [144]. However, it is associated with a high rate of complications, including increased intraocular pressure and cataract development. Around 37% of implanted eyes required surgery to treat glaucoma in a three-year follow-up study. [145]. A cost-effectiveness study showed that the fluocinolone implant was cost-effective compared with systemic immunosuppressive agents in patients with unilateral disease, but not in those requiring bilateral implants. [146].

7.4. Systemic corticosteroids are used in cases of severe bilateral uveitis when topical and/or regional treatment is insufficient to control inflammation, or when systemic disease also requires treatment. A high dose of systemic corticosteroids, such as prednisone 60 mg per day, is generally used for a limited time to avoid ocular and systemic side effects. Prednisone is the most commonly used oral corticosteroid, usually prescribed at a dose of 1 to 1.5 mg/kg/day, then progressively reduced to prevent relapse. In some cases, short-term intravenous administration of methylprednisolone may be used in patients with vision-threatening lesions of the retina or optic nerve, followed by a transition to oral prednisone.

7.5. Systemic immunosuppressive agents are indicated in patients who are corticosteroid-dependent or intolerant. In some cases, a low dose of prednisone, e.g. 5 mg daily, may be preferable to an immunosuppressive agent. Various systemic immunosuppressive drugs have been studied for the treatment of sarcoidosis-related ocular inflammation, such as antimetabolites and calcineurin inhibitors. [147,148,149,150]. The most commonly used drugs for chronic ocular inflammation, including ocular sarcoidosis, include methotrexate, mycophenolate mofetil, azathioprine and ciclosporin. The dosage of these drugs may vary and should be adapted to the specific clinical situation. [152,153,154,155].

The choice of immunosuppressant should be discussed with the patient, taking into account co-morbidities and life plans.

Methotrexate is generally considered the most studied corticosteroid-sparing treatment for sarcoidosis. Studies have demonstrated its efficacy and good tolerability. [152]

Azathioprine is also effective but less well tolerated. [154]

Mycophenolate mofetil (MMF) has been studied to a limited extent, as has cyclosporine. Hydroxychloroquine has shown promising results, but further prospective studies are needed. [153]

Among T-cell inhibitors, cyclosporine and tacrolimus were effective in reducing inflammation in uveitis. Subconjunctival/intravitreal sirolimus showed a dose-dependent benefit (the higher dose was not as effective as a lower dose used in the trial) [45], but is not an FDA-approved option at the time of writing.

7.6. Biological agents, such as tumor necrosis factor (TNF)-a inhibitors, are used as a relatively recent treatment for refractory non-infectious uveitis. Knowledge of their use in ocular conditions is based mainly on case reports, case series and a few non-randomized trials and one double-blind randomized trial. [156]. Biological agents studied to date in the treatment of sarcoidosis-related uveitis include infliximab, adalimumab, etanercept and golimumab.

Infliximab has shown efficacy as an immunosuppressive agent in most patients with refractory uveitis due to a variety of causes. [157]. However, data concerning its specific efficacy in controlling ocular inflammation in sarcoidosis uveitis are limited and mixed. [157,158,159,160]. Some studies have reported an improvement in ocular inflammation in patients with sarcoidosis uveitis after treatment with infliximab, but regular infusions are often required to avoid relapse.

Adalimumab has also been studied as adjunctive therapy in patients with refractory posterior sarcoidosis. In the majority of cases, improvement in intraocular inflammatory signs was observed, including resolution of vasculitis, choroidal involvement, papillitis, macular edema and vitreous haze. [161].

Etanercept is generally considered less effective than infliximab and adalimumab for ocular indications. It showed no significant difference in the control of uveitis associated with juvenile idiopathic arthritis in a randomized trial. [163]. The results of a study on the use of etanercept in refractory sarcoidosis uveitis showed no significant improvement in ocular inflammation compared with placebo. [164].

It is important to note that biological agents may present potential adverse effects and should be used with caution, taking into account the risks and benefits for each individual patient. The decision to use biological agents in the treatment of uveitis should be made in consultation with a specialist in inflammatory diseases of the eye.

Golimumab has been shown to be effective in the treatment of various forms of uveitis in several series of studies. [165,166] For example, Calvo-Rio et al reported successful control of inflammation in two patients with active sarcoid uveitis who had not responded to infliximab. [167] However, follow-up of these patients was limited to 1 and 9 months respectively. Similar results were obtained by Cordero-Coma et al, who studied the use of golimumab in uveitis. Two patients with sarcoidosis uveitis who had not responded to other TNF inhibitors achieved complete control of inflammation after six months of golimumab treatment. [166] Other biotherapies, such as **tocilizumab and Janus kinase (JAK) inhibitors,** have shown promising results in some studies, but their specific use in sarcoid uveitis requires further research.

It should be noted that biologic therapy is currently reserved for secondary or tertiary treatment of sarcoidosis-associated uveitis due to the lack of long-term safety and efficacy data. Although rare, several reports and series suggest that anti-TNF agents such as infliximab, adalimumab, etanercept and certolizumab can cause sarcoidosis-like conditions, including uveitis. [168,169,170,171,172,173]

In the event of initial resistance to corticosteroids and conventional immunosuppressants, other causes such as infectious granulomatosis or lymphoma must be ruled out before considering treatment with biotherapy.

The International Workshop on Ocular Sarcoidosis (IWOS) recommends the following treatment regimen for the management of ocular sarcoidosis [174].

Management of anterior uveitis (AU) in ocular sarcoidosis (OS)

1. Ocular manifestations indicative of UA treatment include anterior chamber (AC) cells, new-onset retrocorneal precipitates, aria nodules, angle nodules, new-onset posterior synechiae and IOP elevation (not induced by corticosteroids).
2. First-line treatment of severe UA (AC cells >3+, new KP, iris nodules) involves instillation of corticosteroid eye drops (prednisolone acetate 1% or similar) at least 10 times a day.
3. The first-line treatment for moderate UA (AC cell <3+) is instillation of a corticosteroid eye drop at least 6 times a day.
4. Second-line treatment for severe UA includes subconjunctival injection of dexamethasone, periocular injection of triamcinolone acetonide and a systemic corticosteroid.
5. Second-line treatment of moderate UA includes more frequent corticosteroid eye drops, a subconjunctival injection of dexamethasone, a periocular injection of triamcinolone acetonide and a systemic corticosteroid.
6. Inactive UA does not require treatment.
7. Mydriatic eye drops are used when UA is active.

Management of intermediate uveitis (IU) in ocular sarcoidosis (OS)

1. Ocular manifestations that indicate treatment in IU include diffuse vitreous opacities, ant-whisk or pack-ice vitreous opacities and macular edema.
2. First-line treatment of active bilateral IU includes a local corticosteroid (periocular, intravitreal, implant) and a systemic corticosteroid.
3. First-line treatment of active unilateral IU is exactly the same as described above.

4. Second-line treatment of active bilateral IU includes a local corticosteroid (periocular, intravitreal, implant), a systemic corticosteroid and non-biological systemic immunosuppressive drugs sparing corticosteroids.

5. Second-line treatment of active unilateral IU is exactly the same as described above.

1.   Ocular manifestations that indicate treatment in UP include macular edema, optic disc nodules/granulomas, nodular and/or segmental periphlebitis, active peripheral chorioretinal lesions and choroidal nodules.

2.   First-line treatment of active bilateral UP includes a systemic corticosteroid alone or combined with non-biological corticosteroid-sparing systemic immunosuppressants and a local corticosteroid (periocular, intravitreal, implant).

3.   First-line treatment of active unilateral UP is exactly the same as described above.

4.   Second-line treatment of active bilateral UP is the same as first-line, with the exception of biologics.

5.   Second-line treatment of active unilateral UP is exactly the same as described above.

1. The average initial dose of systemic prednisone/prednisolone is 0.5-1.0 mg/kg/day, up to a maximum dose of 80 mg/day.

2. The average duration of the initial dose of systemic prednisone/prednisolone is 2 to 4 weeks.

3. The average duration of total treatment with systemic prednisone/prednisolone is 3 to 6 months.

4. Initial corticosteroid-sparing immunosuppressive drugs include methotrexate, azathioprine, mycophenolate mofetil and cyclosporine.

5. In certain cases of severe disease, some specialists may consider administering intravenous corticosteroids.

6. Biological drugs (adalimumab) are used if necessary.

Examples of steroid-based systemic immunosuppressive agents that can be used to treat ocular sarcoidosis

Medicines	Dose	Expected action time
Antimetabolites		
- Methotrexate	7.5-25 mg/week PO, SQ or IM	2-12 weeks
- Mycophenolate mofetil	500-1500 mg PO twice daily	2-12 weeks
- Azathioprine	1-4 mg/kg/day PO daily	4-12 weeks
Calcineurin inhibitors		
- Cyclosporine	2.5-10 mg/kg/day PO twice daily	2-6 weeks
- Tacrolimus	0.15-0.30 mg/kg/day PO	2-6 weeks

IM = intramuscular; PO = oral; SQ = subcutaneous

Adapted from Jabs DA, Rosenbaum JT, Foster CS, Holland GN, Jaffe GJ, Louie JS, Nussenblatt RB, Stiehm ER, Tessler H, Van Gelder RN, Whitcup SM, Yocum D. Guidelines for the use of immunosuppressive drugs in patients with ocular inflammatory disorders: recommendations of an expert panel. *Am J Ophthalmol.* 2000;130(4):492-513; with permi

7.7. Treatment of scleritis and external eye diseases

Non-steroidal anti-inflammatory drugs (NSAIDs) are generally used as first-line treatment for scleritis. If NSAIDs are not effective, corticosteroids are often used. However, concomitant use of NSAIDs and oral corticosteroids can result in significant gastrointestinal adverse effects. In cases where patients fail to respond to or tolerate corticosteroids, systemic immunomodulators may be considered. In one case report, thalidomide was successfully used to treat cutaneous sarcoidosis and nodular scleritis in a patient who had failed to respond to azathioprine and corticosteroids. [175] It should be noted that thalidomide is a controlled drug because of its potential to cause serious birth defects, although it also has anti-inflammatory activity. [176]

In addition to systemic corticosteroid therapy, skin lesions of the eyelids can be treated with intralesional triamcinolone injections or oral chloroquine. [177] Conjunctival lesions and keratoconjunctivitis sicca (KCS) may respond to topical ciclosporin. [178,179]

7.8. Treatment of diseases of the orbit

Treatment of orbital inflammation generally involves the use of oral corticosteroids and/or immunosuppressive agents. In cases where orbital lesions are present or there is a strong suspicion of malignancy, biopsy or removal of the lesions may be necessary. In addition to orbital lesions, problems such as strabismus or abnormal eyelid position may also be observed. It is important to maximize anti-inflammatory treatment first. If surgery is required, orbital surgery should be performed first, followed by strabismus and eyelid surgery, respectively.

7.9 Treatment of ocular complications

It is essential to take into account the treatment of ocular complications that may arise due to ocular inflammation and treatment side effects. Conditions such as glaucoma, cataract, epiretinal membrane formation and cystoid macular edema are common. The use of corticosteroids should be minimized by using other anti-inflammatory agents in patients with elevated intraocular pressure. Cataract surgery can be considered when intraocular inflammation has been stabilized for at least 3 months, to reduce risk. The most important and effective method of treating macular edema is to control intraocular inflammation with anti-inflammatory therapy. [180] In patients whose macular edema persists without active inflammation, intravitreal injections of bevacizumab [181] or ranibizumab [182] have been reported as a possibly effective therapy for improving vision and macular anatomy.

The epiretinal membrane can be surgically removed in those with visually significant folds. However, treatment of associated inflammation and/or edema should be maximized before considering surgery, to avoid postoperative inflammation and unnecessary surgery.

8. Prognosis of ocular sarcoidosis

The visual prognosis of ocular sarcoidosis may vary according to the severity and duration of ocular inflammation, the time to specialist consultation and ocular complications secondary to uveitis. [20] A study investigating the long-term prognosis of sarcoidosis uveitis found that the majority of patients (54%) maintained visual acuity greater than 5/10 in both eyes, and only 4.6% had vision loss of less than 1.6/10 in both eyes, ten years after the onset of uveitis in a specialized ophthalmology center. [183] The main causes of irreversible vision loss were glaucoma and chronic maculopathy linked to inflammation of the posterior segment.

At the onset of uveitis, 35% of the 75 patients had extraocular involvement, and this figure fell to 17% over the following ten years. Approximately 51% of patients required oral corticosteroids and 11% required immunosuppressive drugs for the treatment of uveitis. Around a fifth of patients underwent ocular surgery, such as cataract extraction (17%), trabeculectomy (4%), retinal detachment repair (1%) and epiretinal membrane peeling (1%). The visual prognosis of sarcoidosis uveitis does not appear to be related to the presence of extraocular disease. [183]

In Finland, a study by Karma et al involved 281 patients with biopsy-confirmed sarcoidosis. Of these patients, 21 were followed up regularly because of their uveitis. Of the 21 patients, eight (38%) had a monophasic course of uveitis requiring less than 6 months' treatment, while the remainder (13 patients; 62%) had a recurrent course with several relapses. In the latter group, nine of the 13 patients finally saw their uveitis disappear after several years of treatment. This study also revealed that hilar adenopathy observed on chest X-rays could disappear even if ocular symptoms persisted. This observation suggests that a subgroup of patients with "idiopathic" uveitis may present with sarcoidosis undiagnosed by routine chest radiography. [184]

A study of the 10-year visual prognosis of 69 patients with peripheral multifocal chorioretinitis showed that the presence of systemic sarcoidosis did not influence the risk of developing cystoid macular oedema, epiretinal membrane, cataract, glaucoma or optic atrophy.

Cystoid macular oedema was the main cause of visual impairment. The presence of an epiretinal membrane did not necessarily affect final visual acuity. [185]

It is crucial to inform patients with ocular sarcoidosis that ocular inflammation can be chronic, despite a sudden onset and limited evolution in some cases. Long-term follow-up and strict adherence to treatment are necessary to prevent permanent ocular damage resulting from inflammation and adverse drug reactions.

9. Conclusion

Sarcoidosis is an inflammatory disease that can affect the eyes in 10% to 55% of cases, sometimes without associated systemic involvement. All ocular structures may be affected, but uveitis is the most frequent ocular manifestation, leading to impaired vision. Uveitis generally presents a granulomatous appearance, especially in cases of anterior involvement, often manifesting bilaterally with synechiae formation. Posterior involvement is characterized by vitritis, vasculitis and choroidal lesions. Tuberculosis should be considered a major differential diagnosis, particularly in individuals who have resided in endemic regions. Diagnosis of ocular sarcoidosis is based on histology and the presence of non-caseating epithelioid granulomas, although clinico-radiological features are often used due to technical difficulties and biopsy yields. International diagnostic criteria for ocular sarcoidosis have recently been revised. Corticosteroids remain the first-line treatment for sarcoidosis, but up to 30% of patients require high doses, justifying the use of corticosteroid-sparing therapies. In these cases, immunosuppressive agents such as methotrexate.

Sarcoidosis may require cortisone-sparing therapy, usually with immunosuppressants such as methotrexate, azathioprine, mycophenolate mofetil or cyclosporine. Biological treatments, in particular anti-TNF agents such as adalimumab and infliximab, are used as third-line therapy if conventional treatments fail. Other biotherapies, such as tocilizumab and Janus kinase (JAK) inhibitors, are also being investigated. A multidisciplinary approach and collaboration between specialists are essential to ensure effective management of sarcoidosis uveitis.

References

1. Ungprasert P, Tooley AA, Crowson CS, et al. Clinical characteristics of ocular sarcoidosis: a population-based study 1976-2013. Ocul Immunol Inflamm. 2019;27(3):389-395.

2. Obenauf CD, Shaw HE, Sydnor CF, et al. Sarcoidosis and its ophthalmic manifestations. AmJOphthalmol. 1978;86(5):648-655.

3. Jabs DA, Johns CJ. Ocular involvement in chronic sarcoidosis. Am J Ophthalmol. 1986;102(3): 297-301.

4. Evans, M.; Sharma, O.; LaBree, L.; Smith, R.E.; Rao, N.A. Differences in Clinical Findings between Caucasians and African Americans with Biopsy-Proven Sarcoidosis. *Ophthalmology* **2007**,*114*, 325-333. [CrossRef] [PubMed]

5. Jamilloux, Y.; Kodjikian, L.; Broussolle, C.; Sève, P. Sarcoidosis and uveitis. *Autoimmun. Rev.* **2014**,*13*, 840-849. [CrossRef]

6. Ungprasert, P.; Tooley, A.A.; Crowson, C.S.; Matteson, E.L.; Smith, W.M. Clinical features of ocular sarcoidosis: A population-based study 1976-2013. *Ocul. Immunol. Inflamm.* **2019**, *27*, 389-395. [CrossRef]

7. Tsirouki, T.; Dastiridou, A.; Symeonidis, C.; Tounakaki, O.; Brazitikou, I.; Kalogeropoulos, C.; Androudi, S. Focus on the epidemiology of uveitis. *Ocul. Immunol. Inflamm.* **2018**, *26*, 2-16. [CrossRef]

8. Arkema, E.V.; Cozier, Y.C. Epidemiology of sarcoidosis: Recent estimates of incidence, prevalence and risk factors. *Curr. Opin. Pulm. Med.* **2020**, *26*, 527-534. [CrossRef]

9. Baughman, R.P.; Field, S.; Costabel, U.; Crystal, R.G.; Culver, D.A.; Drent, M.; Judson, M.A.; Wolff, G. Sarcoidosis in America. An analysis based on health care utilization. *Ann. Am. Thorac. Soc.* **2016**,*13*, 1244-1252. [CrossRef]

10. Duchemann, B.; Annesi-Maesano, I.; Jacobe de Naurois, C.; Sanyal, S.; Brillet, P.-Y.; Brauner, M.; Kambouchner, M.; Huynh, S.; Naccache, J.M.; Borie, R.; et al. Prevalence and Incidence of Interstitial Lung Diseases in a Multi-Ethnic County of Greater Paris. *Eur. Respir. J.* **2017**, *50*, 1602419. [CrossRef] [PubMed]

11. Cardoso, A.V.; Mota, P.C.; Melo, N.; Guimaraes, S.; Souto Moura, C.; Jesus, J.M.; Cunha, R.; Morais, A. Analysis of sarcoidosis in the Porto region (Portugal). *Rev. Port. Pneumol.* **2017**, *23*, 251-258. [CrossRef] [PubMed]

12. Crick, R.P.; Hoyle, C.; Smellie, H. THE EYES IN SARCOIDOSIS. *Br. J. Ophthalmol.* **1961**, *45*, 461-481. [CrossRef]

13. Morimoto, T.; Azuma, A.; Abe, S.; Usuki, J.; Kudoh, S.; Sugisaki, K.; Oritsu, M.; Nukiwa, T. Epidemiology of sarcoidosis in Japan. *Eur. Respir. J.* **2008**, *31*, 372-379. [CrossRef]

14. Kitamei, H.; Kitaichi, N.; Namba, K.; Kotake, S.; Goda, C.; Kitamura, M.; Miyazaki, A.; Ohno, S. Clinical features of intraocular inflammation in Hokkaido, Japan. *Acta Ophthalmol.* **2009**, *87*, 424-428. [CrossRef]

15. A. Ocular involvement in sarcoidosis. Br J Ophthalmol. 2000; 84(1):110-116. [PubMed: 10611110]

16. Ohara K, Okubo A, Sasaki H, Kamata K. Intraocular manifestations of systemic sarcoidosis. Jpn J Ophthalmol. 1992; 36(4):452-457. [PubMed: 1289622]

17. Heiligenhaus A, Wefelmeyer D, Wefelmeyer E, Rosel M, Schrenk M. The eye as a common site for the early clinical manifestation of sarcoidosis. Ophthalmic Res. 2011; 46(1):9-12. [PubMed: 21099232]

18. Rothova A, Alberts C, Glasius E, Kijlstra A, Buitenhuis HJ, Breebaart AC. Risk factors for ocular sarcoidosis. Doc Ophthalmol. 1989; 72(3-4):287-296. [PubMed: 2625091]

19. Hoover DL, Khan JA, Giangiacomo J. Pediatric ocular sarcoidosis. Surv Ophthalmol. 1986; 30(4): 215-228. [PubMed: 3006270]

20. Rose CD, Wouters CH, Meiorin S, Doyle TM, Davey MP, Rosenbaum JT, Martin TM. Pediatric granulomatous arthritis: an international registry. Arthritis Rheum. 2006; 54(10):3337-3344. [PubMed: 17009307]

21. Dana MR, Merayo-Lloves J, Schaumberg DA, Foster CS. Prognosticatorsforvisual outcome in sarcoid uveitis. Ophthalmology. 1996; 103(11):1846-1853. [PubMed: 8942880]

22. Evans M, Sharma O, LaBree L, Smith RE, Rao NA. Differences in clinical findings between Caucasians and African Americans with biopsy-proven sarcoidosis. Ophthalmology. 2007; 114(2): 325-333. [PubMed: 17123620]

23. Birnbaum AD, Oh FS, Chakrabarti A, Tessler HH, Goldstein DA. Clinical features and diagnostic evaluation of biopsy-proven ocular sarcoidosis. Arch Ophthalmol. 2011; 129(4):409-413. [PubMed: 21482866]

24. Kump LI, Cervantes-Castaneda RA, Androudi SN, Foster CS. Analysis of pediatric uveitis cases at a tertiary referral center. Ophthalmology. 2005; 112(7):1287-1292. [PubMed: 15921752]

25. Smith JA, Mackensen F, Sen HN, Leigh JF, Watkins AS, Pyatetsky D, Tessler HH, Nussenblatt RB, Rosenbaum JT, Reed GF, Vitale S, Smith JR, Goldstein DA. Epidemiology and course of disease in childhood uveitis. Ophthalmology. 2009; 116(8):1544-1551. 1551 e1541. [PubMed: 19651312]

26. Rodriguez A, Calonge M, Pedroza-Seres M, Akova YA, Messmer EM, D'Amico DJ, Foster CS. Referral patterns of uveitis in a tertiary eye care center. Arch Ophthalmol. 1996; 114(5):593-599. [PubMed: 8619771]

27. Merrill PT, Kim J, Cox TA, Betor CC, McCallum RM, Jaffe GJ. Uveitis in the southeastern United States. Curr Eye Res. 1997; 16(9):865-874. [PubMed: 9288447]

28. Sungur G, Hazirolan D, Bilgin G. Pattern of ocular findings in patients with biopsy- proven sarcoidosis in Turkey. Ocul Immunol Inflamm. 2013; 21(6):455-461. [PubMed: 23909887]

29. Abad S, Meyssonier V, Allali J, Gouya H, Giraudet AL, Monnet D, Parc C, Tenenbaum F, Alberini JL, Grabar S, Pesce F, Rollot F, Sicard D, Dhote R, Blanche P, Brezin AP. Association of peripheral multifocal choroiditis with sarcoidosis: a study of thirty- seven patients. Arthritis Rheum. 2004; 51(6):974-982. [PubMed: 15593175]

30. Ossewaarde-van Norel J, Ten Dam-van Loon N, de Boer JH, Rothova A. Long-term visual prognosis of peripheral multifocal chorioretinitis. Am J Ophthalmol. 2015; 159(4):690-697. [PubMed: 25595670]

31. Rossman MD, Thompson B, Frederick M, Maliarik M, Iannuzzi MC, Rybicki BA, Pandey JP, Newman LS, Magira E, Beznik-Cizman B, Monos D, Group A. HLA-DRB1*1101: a significant risk factor for sarcoidosis in blacks and whites. Am J Hum Genet. 2003; 73(4):720-735. [PubMed: 14508706]

32. Rothova, A.; Alberts, C.; Glasius, E.; Kijlstra, A.; Buitenhuis, H.J.; Breebaart, A.C. Risk factors for ocular sarcoidosis. *Doc. Ophthalmol.* **1989**,

33. Febvay, C.; Kodjikian, L.; Maucort-Boulch, D.; Perard, L.; Iwaz, J.; Jamilloux, Y.; Broussolle, C.; Burillon, C.; Seve, P. Clinical features and diagnostic evaluation of 83 biopsy-proven cases of sarcoidosis uveitis. *Br. J. Ophthalmol.* **2015**,

34. Fermon, C.; El-Jammal, T.; Kodjikian, L.; Burillon, C.; Hot, A.; Pérard, L.; Mathis, T.; Jamilloux, Y.; Sève, P. Identification of Multidimensional Phenotypes Using Cluster Analysis in Sarcoid Uveitis Patients. *Am. J. Ophthalmol.* **2022**,

35. Schupp, J.C.; Freitag-Wolf, S.; Bargagli, E.; Mihailovic'-Vuc "inic', V.; Rottoli, P.; Grubanovic, A.; Müller, A.; Jochens, A.; Tittmann, L.; Schnerch, J.; et al. Phenotypes of Organ Involvement in Sarcoidosis. *Eur. Respir. J.* **2018**, *51*,

36. Van Swol, J.M.; Hawkins, E.T.; Joseph, E.D.; Nguyen, S.A.; Anderson, R.J.; Thompson, E.B.; Perry, L.J.; Sandhu, H.S. Cardiac Screening and Disease Characteristics of Patients with Ocular Sarcoidosis. *Ocul. Immunol. Inflamm.* **2022**;

37. Richard, M.; Jamilloux, Y.; Courand, P.-Y.; Perard, L.; Durel, C.-A.; Hot, A.; Burillon, C.; Durieu, I.; Gerfaud-Valentin, M.; Kodjikian, L.; et al. Cardiac Sarcoidosis Is Uncommon in Patients with Isolated Sarcoid Uveitis: Outcome of 294 Cases. *J. Clin. Med.* **2021**,

38. Niederer, R.L.; Ma, S.P.; Wilsher, M.L.; Ali, N.Q.; Sims, J.L.; Tomkins-Netzer, O.; Lightman, S.L.; Lim, L.L. Systemic associations of sarcoidosis uveitis : Correlation with uveitis phenotype and ethnicity. *Am. J. Ophthalmol.* **2021**,

39. Sonoda KH, Hasegawa E, Namba K, JOIS (Japanese Ocular Inflammation Society) Uveitis Survey Working Group, et al. Epidemiology of uveitis in Japan: a 2016 retrospective nationwide survey. Jpn J Ophthalmol. 2021

40. Uveitis Nomenclature Standardization Working Group (SUN) Development of classification criteria for uveitis. *Am. J. Ophthalmol.* **2021**,

41. Baughman, R.P.; Teirstein, A.S.; Judson, M.A.; Rossman, M.D.; Yeager, H.; Bresnitz, E.A.; DePalo, L.; Hunninghake, G.; Iannuzzi, M.C.; Johns, C.J.; et al. Clinical characteristics of patients in a case-control study of sarcoidosis. *Am. J. Respir. Crit. Care Med.* **2001**,

42. Ma, S.P.; Rogers, S.L.; Hall, A.J.; Hodgson, L.; Brennan, J.; Stawell, R.J.; Lim, L.L. Sarcoidosis-Related Uveitis: Clinical presentation, disease course, and rate of progression of systemic disease after diagnosis of uveitis. *Am. J. Ophthalmol.* **2019**

43. Birnbaum, A.D.; French, D.D.; Mirsaeidi, M.; Wehrli, S. Sarcoidosis in the national veteran population: Association of ocular inflammation and mortality. *Ophthalmology* **2015**,

44. Rochepeau, C.; Jamilloux, Y.; Kerever, S.; Febvay, C.; Perard, L.; Broussolle, C.; Burillon, C.; Kodjikian, L.; Seve, P. Long-Term Visual and Systemic Prognoses of 83 Cases of Biopsy-Proven Sarcoid Uveitis. *Br. J. Ophthalmol.* **2017**

45. Reid, G.; Williams, M.; Compton, M.; Silvestri, G.; McAvoy, C. Ocular Sarcoidosis Prevalence and Clinical Features in the Northern Ireland Population. *Eye* **2022**,

46. Coulon, C.; Kodjikian, L.; Rochepeau, C.; Perard, L.; Jardel, S.; Burillon, C.; Broussolle, C.; Jamilloux, Y.; Seve, P. Ethnicity and association with ocular and systemic manifestations and prognosis in 194 patients with sarcoidosis uveitis. *Graefes Arch. Clin. Exp. Ophthalmol.* **2019**,

47. Uveitis nomenclature standardization (SUN) working group classification criteria for sarcoidosis-associated uveitis. *Am. J. Ophthalmol.* **2021**,

48. Mochizuki, M.; Smith, J.R.; Takase, H.; Kaburaki, T.; Acharya, N.R.; Rao, N.A.; International Workshop on Ocular Sarcoidosis Study Group. Revised International Workshop on Ocular Sarcoidosis (IWOS) criteria for the diagnosis of ocular sarcoidosis. *Br. J. Ophthalmol.* **2019**,

49. Crouser, E.D.; Maier, L.A.; Wilson, K.C.; Bonham, C.A.; Morgenthau, A.S.; Patterson, K.C.; Abston, E.; Bernstein, R.C.; Blankstein, R.; Chen, E.S.; et al. Diagnosis and detection of sarcoidosis. An Official American Thoracic Society Clinical Practice Guideline. *Am. J. Respir. Crit. Care Med.* **2020**,

50. Lee, J.; Zaguia, F.; Minkus, C.; Koreishi, A.F.; Birnbaum, A.D.; Goldstein, D.A. The Role of Screening for Asymptomatic Ocular Inflammation in Sarcoidosis. *Ocul. Immunol. Inflamm.* **2022**, *30*,

51. Jabs, D.A.; Nussenblatt, R.B.; Rosenbaum, J.T.; Standardization of Uveitis Nomenclature (SUN) Working Group Standardization of Uveitis Nomenclature for Reporting Clinical Data. Results of the first international workshop. *Am. J. Ophthalmol.* **2005,**

52. Edelsten, C.; Pearson, A.; Joynes, E.; Stanford, M.R.; Graham, E.M. The Ocular and Systemic Prognosis of Patients Presenting with Sarcoid Uveitis. *Eye* **1999,**

53. Grumet, P.; Kerever, S.; Gilbert, T.; Kodjikian, L.; Gerfaud-Valentin, M.; De Parisot, A.; Jamilloux, Y.; Sève, P. Clinical and etiological features of de novo uveitis in patients aged 60 and over: Experience from a French tertiary center. *Graefes Arch. Clin. Exp. Ophthalmol.* **2019,**

54. Classification criteria for pars planitis from the working group on standardization of uveitis nomenclature (SUN). *Am. J. Ophthalmol.* **2021,**

55. Bertrand, P.-J.; Jamilloux, Y.; Ecochard, R.; Richard-Colmant, G.; Gerfaud-Valentin, M.; Guillaud, M.; Denis, P.; Kodjikian, L.; Sève, P. Uveitis: Autoimmunity ... and beyond. *Autoimmun. Rev.* **2019,**

56. Ness, T.; Boehringer, D.; Heinzelmann, S. Intermediate uveitis: Model of etiology, complications, treatment and outcomes in a tertiary academic center. *Orphanet. J. Rare Dis.* **2017,** *12,* 81. [CrossRef]

57. Jones, N.P. The Manchester Uveitis Clinic: The First 3000 Patients-Epidemiology and Casemix. *Ocul. Immunol. Inflamm.* **2015,** *23,* 118-126. [CrossRef]

58. Heiligenhaus, A.; Wefelmeyer, D.; Wefelmeyer, E.; Rosel, M.; Schrenk, M. The Eye as a Common Site for the Early Clinical Manifestation of Sarcoidosis. *Ophthalmic Res.* **2011,** *46,* 9-12. [CrossRef]

59. Dana, M.R.; Merayo-Lloves, J.; Schaumberg, D.A.; Foster, C.S. Prognosticators for Visual Outcome in Sarcoid Uveitis. *Ophthalmology* **1996,** *103,* 1846-1853. [CrossRef].

60. Hage, D.G.; Wahab, C.H.; Kheir, W.J. Choroidal sarcoidal granuloma: A Case Report and Review of the Literature. *J. Ophthalmic Inflamm. Infect.* **2022,** *12,* 31 [CrossRef] [PubMed]

61. Oyeniran, E.; Katz, D.; Kodati, S. Isolated Optic Disc Granuloma as a Presenting Sign of Sarcoidosis. *Ocul. Immunol. Inflamm.* 2022; *in press.* [CrossRef]

62. de Saint Sauveur, G.; Gratiot, C.; Debieb, A.C.; Monnet, D.; Brézin, A.P. Retinal and preretinal nodules: A rare manifestation of probable ocular sarcoidosis. *Am. J. Ophthalmol. Case Rep.* **2022**, *26*, 101525. [CrossRef] [PubMed]

63. Campo, R.V.; Aaberg, T.M. Choroidal Granuloma in Sarcoidosis. *Am. J. Ophthalmol.* **1984**, *97*, 419-427. [CrossRef] [PubMed]

64. Cerquaglia, A.; Iaccheri, B.; Fiore, T.; Fruttini, D.; Belli, F.B.; Khairallah, M.; Lupidi, M.; Cagini, C. New perspectives on ocular sarcoidosis: An Optical Coherence Tomography Angiography Study. *Ocul. Immunol. Inflamm.* **2019**,

65. Hiroshi Takase (2021): Characteristics and management of ocular sarcoidosis, Immunological Medicine, DOI: 10.1080/25785826.2021.1940740

66. Usui, Y.; Goto, H. Granuloma-like Formation in Deeper Retinal Plexus in Ocular Sarcoidosis. *Clin. Ophthalmol.* **2019**

67. Rothova, A. Ocular Involvement in Sarcoidosis. *Br. J. Ophthalmol.* **2000**, *84*, 110-116. [CrossRef] [PubMed]

68. Lezrek, O.; El Kaddoumi, M.; Cherkaoui, O. "Candle Wax Dripping" Lesions in Sarcoidosis. *JAMA Ophthalmol.* **2017**,*135*, e171845. [CrossRef]

69. Fajnkuchen, F.; Badelon, I.; Battesti, J.P.; Valeyre, D.; Chaine, G. Retinal vasculature in sarcoidosis. *Presse Med.* **2000**, *29*, 1801-1806.

70. Vongkulsiri, S.; Vanichseni, S.; Choontanom, R.; Keorochana, N. Characteristics, etiology and clinical outcomes of retinal vasculitis in a tertiary hospital in Thailand. *Ocul. Immunol. Inflamm.* 2023; *in press.* [CrossRef]

71. Giorgiutti, S.; Jacquot, R.; El Jammal, T.; Bert, A.; Jamilloux, Y.; Kodjikian, L.; Sève, P. Sarcoidosis- Related Uveitis: A Review. *J. Clin. Med.***2023**,*12*,3194. https://doi.org/ 10.3390/jcm12093194

72. Zaidi, A.A.; Ying, G.-S.; Daniel, E.; Gangaputra, S.; Rosenbaum, J.T.; Suhler, E.B.; Thorne, J.E.; Foster, C.S.; Jabs, D.A.; Levy-Clarke,

G.A.; et al. Hypopyon in Patients with Uveitis. *Ophthalmology* **2010**,*117*, 366-372. [CrossRef]

73. Ohguro, N.; Sonoda, K.-H.; Takeuchi, M.; Matsumura, M.; Mochizuki, M. The 2009 Prospective Multi-Center Epidemiologic Survey of Uveitis in Japan. *Jpn. J. Ophthalmol.* **2012**, *56*, 432-435. [CrossRef]

74. Lobo, A.; Barton, K.; Minassian, D.; du Bois, R.M.; Lightman, S. Visual loss in sarcoidal uveitis. *Clin. Exp. Ophthalmol.* **2003**,

75. Delaney P. Neurologic manifestations in sarcoidosis: review ofthe literature, with a report of 23 cases. Ann Intern Med. 1977; 87(3):336-345. [PubMed: 197863]

76. Phillips YL, Eggenberger ER. Neuro-ophthalmic sarcoidosis. Curr Opin Ophthalmol. 2010; 21(6): 423-429. [PubMed: 20736834]

77. GassJD, Olson CL. Sarcoidosis with optic nerve and retinal involvement. Arch Ophthalmol. 1976; 94(6):945-950. [PubMed: 938285]

78. Zajicek JP, Scolding NJ, Foster O, Rovaris M, Evanson J, Moseley IF, Scadding JW, Thompson EJ, Chamoun V, Miller DH, McDonald WI, Mitchell D. Central nervous system sarcoidosis-- diagnosis and management. QJM. 1999; 92(2):103-117. [PubMed: 10209662]

79. Oie K, Tanigawa K, Suganuma Y, Matsushima Y, Inaba Y. [A case of CNS sarcoidosis - case report of hydrocephalus due to mechanical obstruction secondary to sarcoid granulomata at the outlet ofthe fourth ventricle (author's transl)]. No Shinkei Geka. 1981; 9(1):75-78. [PubMed: 7231630]

80. Zhang J, Waisbren E, Hashemi N, Lee AG. Visual hallucinations (Charles Bonnet syndrome) associated with neurosarcoidosis. Middle East Afr J Ophthalmol. 2013; 20(4):369-371. [PubMed: 24339694]

81. Yaosaka M, Abe R, Ujiie H, Abe Y, Shimizu H. Unilateral periorbital oedema due to sarcoid infiltration ofthe eyelid: an unusual presentation of sarcoidosis with facial nerve palsy and parotid gland enlargement. Br J Dermatol. 2007; 157(l):200-202. [PubMed: 17489978]

82. Pessoa de Souza Filho J, Martins MC, Sant'Anna AE, Coutinho AB, Burnier MN Jr. Rigueiro MP. Eyelid swelling as the only manifestation of ocularsarcoidosis. Ocul Immunol Inflamm. 2005; 13(5):399-402. [PubMed: 16419426]

83. Hall JG, Cohen KL. Sarcoidosis of the eyelid skin. Am J Ophthalmol. 1995; 119(1):100- 101. [PubMed:7825675]

84. Kim YJ, Kim YD. A case of scar sarcoidosis of the eyelid. Korean J Ophthalmol. 2006; 20(4):238- 240 [PubMed: 17302211].

85. Papadaki TG, Kafkala C, Zacharopoulos IP, Seyedahmadi BJ, Dryja T, Foster CS. Conjunctival non-caseating granulomas in a human immunodeficiency virus (HIV) positive patient attributed to sarcoidosis. Ocul Immunol Inflamm. 2006; 14(5):309- 311. [PubMed: 17056466]

86. Manrique Lipa RK, de los Bueis AB, De los Rios JJ, Manrique Lipa RD. Sarcoidosis presenting as acute bulbar follicular conjunctivitis. Clin Exp Optom. 2010; 93(5):363- 365. [PubMed: 20718787]

87. Dursun D, Akova YA, Bilezikci B. Scleritis associated with sarcoidosis. Ocul Immunol Inflamm. 2004; 12(2):143-148. [PubMed: 15512984]

88. Babu K, Kini R, Mehta R. Scleral nodule and bilateral disc edema as a presenting manifestation of systemic sarcoidosis. Ocul Immunol Inflamm. 2010; 18(3):158-161. [PubMed: 20482388]

89. Dodds EM, LowderCY, Barnhorst DA, Lavertu P, Caravella LP, White DE. Posterior scleritis with annular ciliochoroidal detachment. Am J Ophthalmol. 1995; 120(5):677- 679 [PubMed:7485375].

90. Riono WP, Hidayat AA, Rao NA. Scleritis: a clinicopathologic study of 55 cases. Ophthalmology. 1999; 106(7):1328-1333. [PubMed: 10406616]

91. Lennarson P, Barney NP. Interstitial keratitis as presenting ophthalmic sign of sarcoidosis in a child. J Pediatr Ophthalmol Strabismus. 1995; 32(3):194-196. [PubMed:7636703]

92. Siracuse-Lee D, Saffra N. Peripheral ulcerative keratitis in sarcoidosis: a case report. Cornea. 2006

93. Mavrikakis I, Rootman J. Diverse clinical presentations of orbital sarcoid. Am J Ophthalmol. 2007

94. Demirci H, Christianson MD. Orbital and adnexal involvement in sarcoidosis: analysis of clinical features and systemic disease in 30 cases. Am J Ophthalmol. 2011

95. Jones BR, Stevenson CJ. Keratoconjunctivitis sicca due to sarcoidosis. Br J Ophthalmol. 1957;

96. Chapman KL, Bartley GB, Garrity JA, Gonnering RS. Lacrimal bypass surgery in patients with sarcoidosis. Am J Ophthalmol. 1999;

97. Kay DJ, Saffra N, Har-El G. Isolated sarcoidosis of the lacrimal sac without systemic manifestations. Am J Otolaryngol. 2002

98. Prabhakaran VC, Saeed P, Esmaeli B, Sullivan TJ, McNab A, Davis G, Valenzuela A, Leibovitch I, Kesler A, Sivak-Callcott J, Hoyama E, Selva D. Orbital and adnexal sarcoidosis. Arch Ophthalmol. 2007

99. Kim DS, Korgavkar K, Zahid S, De Lott L, Prabhakar A, Foerster BR, Besirli CG. Vision Loss After Central Retinal Artery Occlusion Secondary to Orbital Sarcoid Mass. Ophthal Plast Reconstr Surg. 2014

100. Jabs DA, Johns CJ. Ocular involvement in chronic sarcoidosis. Am J Ophthalmol. 1986;

101. Shimizu A, Maruyama K, Yokoyama Y, Tsuda S, Ryu M, Nakazawa T. Characteristics of uveitic glaucoma and evaluation of its surgical treatment. Clin Ophthalmol. 2014

102. Sève, P.; Cacoub, P.; Bodaghi, B.; Trad, S.; Sellam, J.; Bellocq, D.; Bielefeld, P.; Sène, D.; Kaplanski, G.; Monnet, D.; et al. Uveitis: Diagnostic Work-up. Review of the literature and recommendations of an expert committee. *Autoimmun. Rev.* **2017**, *16*, 1254-1264. [CrossRef] [PubMed]

103. Akpek, E.K.; Ahmed, I.; Hochberg, F.H.; Soheilian, M.; Dryja, T.P.; Jakobiec, F.A.; Foster, C.S. Intraocular-Central Nervous System Lymphoma: Clinical features, diagnosis and outcome. *Ophthalmology* **1999**,*106*, 1805-1810. [CrossRef].

104. Cowan, C.L. Disease review of the year: Differential Diagnosis of Ocular Sarcoidosis. *Ocul. Immunol. Inflamm.* **2010**,*18*, 442-451. [CrossRef] [PubMed]

105. Mehta, S.; Peters, R.P.; Smit, D.P.; Gupta, V. Ocular tuberculosis in HIV-infected individuals. *Ocul. Immunol. Inflamm.* **2020**, *28*, 1251-1258. [CrossRef] [PubMed]

106. Babu, K.; Biswas, J.; Agarwal, M.; Mahendradas, P.; Bansal, R.; Rathinam, S.R.; Basu, S.; Ganesh, S.K.; Konana, V.K.; Vedhanayaki, R.; et al. Diagnostic Markers in Ocular Sarcoidosis in A High TB Endemic Population-A Multicentre Study. *Ocul. Immunol. Inflamm.* **2022**, *30*, 163-167. [CrossRef] [PubMed]

107. Heinle, R.; Chang, C. Diagnostic criteria for sarcoidosis. *Autoimmun. Rev.* **2014**, *13*, 383-387. [CrossRef] [PubMed]

108. Crick, R.; Hoyle, C.; Mather, G. Conjunctival biopsy in sarcoidosis. *Br. Med. J.* **1955**, *2*, 1180-1181. [CrossRef].

109. Zina, S.; Khairallah, M.; Ben Amor, H.; Ksiaa, I.; Hadhri, R.; Attia, S.; Khochtali, S.; Khairallah, M. Conjunctival granulomas leading to the diagnosis of systemic sarcoidosis. *J. Fr. Ophthalmol.* **2022**, *45*, e67-e69. [CrossRef]

110. Papadaki TG, Kafkala C, Zacharopoulos IP, Seyedahmadi BJ, Dryja T, Foster CS. Conjunctival non-caseating granulomas in a human immunodeficiency virus (HIV) positive patient attributed to sarcoidosis. Ocul Immunol Inflamm. 2006; 14(5):309- 311. [PubMed: 17056466]

111. Manrique Lipa RK, de los Bueis AB, De los Rios JJ, Manrique Lipa RD. Sarcoidosis presenting as acute bulbar follicular conjunctivitis. Clin Exp Optom. 2010; 93(5):363-365. [PubMed: 20718787]

112. Grumet, P.; Kodjikian, L.; de Parisot, A.; Errera, M.-H.; Sedira, N.; Heron, E.; Pérard, L.; Cornut, P.-L.; Schneider, C.; Rivière, S.; et al. Contribution des tests diagnostiques au bilan étiologique des uvéites, données de l'étude ULISSE (Uveitis: Évaluation clinique et médico-économique d'une stratégie standardisée du diagnostic étiologique). *Autoimmun. Rev.* **2018**,

113. Avendano-Monje, C.L.; Cordero-Coma, M.; Mauriz, J.L.; Calleja-Antolin, S.; Fonollosa, A.; Garrote Llordén, A.; Martin Garcia-Sancho, J.; Sanchez-Salazar, M.I.; Ruiz de Morales, J.G. Anti-Retinal Antibodies in Sarcoidosis. *Ocul. Immunol. Inflamm.* 2022

114. Gundlach, E.; Hoffmann, M.M.; Prasse, A.; Heinzelmann, S.; Ness, T. Interleukin-2 Receptor and Angiotensin-Converting Enzyme as Markers for Ocular Sarcoidosis. *PLoS ONE* **2016**, *11*, e0147258. [CrossRef]

115. Bennett, D.; Cameli, P.; Lanzarone, N.; Carobene, L.; Bianchi, N.; Fui, A.; Rizzi, L.; Bergantini, L.; Cillis, G.; d'Alessandro, M.; et al. Chitotriosidase: A Biomarker of Activity and Severity in Patients with Sarcoidosis. *Respir. Res.* **2020**,

116. Birnbaum, A.D.; Oh, F.S.; Chakrabarti, A.; Tessler, H.H.; Goldstein, D.A. Clinical Features and Diagnostic Evaluation of BiopsyProven Ocular Sarcoidosis. *Arch. Ophthalmol.* **2011,**

117. Zhang, Y.; Du, S.-S.; Zhao, M.-M.; Li, Q.-H.; Zhou, Y.; Song, J.-C.; Chen, T.; Shi, J.-Y.; Jie, B.; Li, W.; et al. Chest High-Resolution Computed Tomography Can Make Higher Accurate Stages for Thoracic Sarcoidosis than X-Ray. *BMCPulm. Med.* **2022,**

118. Vender, R.J.; Aldahham, H.; Gupta, R. The role of PET in the management of sarcoidosis. *Curr. Opin. Pulm. Med.* **2022,**

119. Nishiyama, Y.; Yamamoto, Y.; Fukunaga, K.; Takinami, H.; Iwado, Y.; Satoh, K.; Ohkawa, M. Comparative Evaluation of 18F-FDG PET and 67Ga Scintigraphy in Patients with Sarcoidosis. *J. Nucl. Med.* **2006,**

120. Rahmi, A.; Deshayes, E.; Maucort-Boulch, D.; Varron, L.; Grange, J.D.; Kodjikian, L.; Seve, P. Intraocular sarcoidosis: Association of clinical features of uveitis with 18F-labelled fluorodeoxyglucose positron emission tomography findings. *Br. J. Ophthalmol.* **2012,**

121. Chauvelot, P.; Skanjeti, A.; Jamilloux, Y.; de Parisot, A.; Broussolle, C.; Denis, P.; Ramackers, J.M.; Giammarile, F.; Kodjikian, L.; Seve, P. 18F-Fluorodeoxyglucose Positron Emission Tomography Is Useful for the Diagnosis of Intraocular Sarcoidosis in Patients with a Normal CT Scan. *Br. J. Ophthalmol.* **2019,**

122. Burger, C.; Holness, J.L.; Smit, D.P.; Griffith-Richards, S.; Koegelenberg, C.F.N.; Ellmann, A. The Role of 18F-FDG PET/CT in Suspected Intraocular Sarcoidosis and Tuberculosis. *Ocul. Immunol. Inflamm.* **2021,**

123. Sahin, 0.; Ziaei, A.; Karaismailog "lu, E.; Taheri, N. The Serum Angiotensin Converting Enzyme and Lysozyme Levels in Patients with Ocular Involvement of Autoimmune and Infectious Diseases. BMC Ophthalmol. 2016

124. Takahashi, T.; Azuma, A.; Abe, S.; Kawanami, O.; Ohara, K.; Kudoh, S. Significance of Lymphocytosis in Bronchoalveolar Lavage in Suspected Ocular Sarcoidosis. *Eur. Respir. J.* **2001,**

125. Maruyama, K.; Inaba, T.; Tamada, T.; Nakazawa, T. Vitreous Lavage Fluid and Bronchoalveolar Lavage Fluid Have Equal Diagnostic Value in Sarcoidosis. *Medicine (Baltimore)* **2016**,

126. Kojima, K.; Maruyama, K.; Inaba, T.; Nagata, K.; Yasuhara, T.; Yoneda, K.; Sugita, S.; Mochizuki, M.; Kinoshita, S. The CD4/CD8 Ratio in Vitreous Fluid Is of High Diagnostic Value in Sarcoidosis. Ophthalmology 2012,

127. De Simone, L.; Bonacini, M.; Aldigeri, R.; Alessandrello, F.; Mastrofilippo, V.; Gozzi, F.; Bolletta, E.; Adani, C.; Zerbini, A.; Cavallini, G.M.; et al. Can different cytokine profiles in aqueous humor and plasma help differentiate ocular diseases? Sarcoidosis and ocular tuberculosis? *Inflamm. Res.* **2022**,

128. Komatsu, H.; Usui, Y.; Tsubota, K.; Fujii, R.; Yamaguchi, T.; Maruyama, K.; Wakita, R.; Asakage, M.; Shimizu, H.; Yamakawa, N.; et al. Comprehensive Proteomic Profiling of Vitreous Humor in Ocular Sarcoidosis Compared with Other Vitreoretinal Diseases. J. Clin. Med. 2022,

129. Blaise, P.; Fardeau, C.; Chapelon, C.; Bodaghi, B.; Le Hoang, P. Minor Salivary Gland Biopsy in Diagnosing Ocular Sarcoidosis. Br. J. Ophthalmol. 2011,

130. Bernard, C.; Kodjikian, L.; Bancel, B.; Isaac, S.; Broussolle, C.; Seve, P. Ocular sarcoidosis: When should a labial salivary gland biopsy be performed? Graefes Arch. Clin. Exp. Ophthalmol. 2013,

131. Crombag, L.M.M.; Mooij-Kalverda, K.; Szlubowski, A.; Gnass, M.; Tournoy, K.G.; Sun, J.; Oki, M.; Ninaber, M.K.; Steinfort, D.P.; Jennings, B.R.; et al. EBUS versus EUS-B for Diagnosing Sarcoidosis: The International Sarcoidosis Assessment (ISA) Randomized Clinical Trial. Respirology 2022,

132. Sudheer, B.; Agarwal, M.; Sharma, D.; Mehta, R.; Babu, K. Role of Endobronchial Ultrasound Guided Transbronchial Needle Aspiration in the Diagnosis of Intraocular Inflammation in India-Our Experience. Ocul. Immunol. Inflamm. 2019,

133. Suzuki, K.; Ishihara, M.; Namba, K.; Ohno, S.; Goto, H.; Takase, H.; Kawano, S.; Shibuya, E.; Hase, K.; Iwata, D.; et al. Clinical Characteristics of ocular sarcoidosis: Severe, refractory and prolonged inflammation. Jpn. J. Ophthalmol. 2022, 66, 447-454. [CrossRef]

134. Groen, F.; Rothova, A. Ocular involvement in sarcoidosis. Semin. Respir. Crit. Care Med. 2017, 38, 514-522. [CrossRef]

135. Paovic, J.; Paovic, P.; Sredovic, V.; Jovanovic, S. Clinical manifestations, complications and treatment of ocular sarcoidosis: Correlation between Visual Efficiency and Macular Edema as Seen on Optical Coherence Tomography. In Seminars in Ophthalmology; Taylor & Francis: New York, NY, USA, 2016

136. Nagahori, K.; Keino, H.; Nakayama, M.; Watanabe, T.; Ando, Y.; Hayashi, I.; Abe, S.; Okada, A.A. Clinical features and visual outcomes of ocular sarcoidosis in a tertiary referral center in Tokyo. *Graefes Arch. Clin. Exp. Ophthalmol.* **2022**,

137. Stavrou, P.; Linton, S.; Young, D.W.; Murray, P.I. Clinical diagnosis of ocular sarcoidosis. *Eye* **1997**,

138. Bienvenu, F.-H.; Tiffet, T.; Maucort-Boulch, D.; Gerfaud-Valentin, M.; Kodjikian, L.; Perard, L.; Burillon, C.; Durel, C.-A.; Hot, A.; Jamilloux, Y.; et al. Factors Associated with Ocular and Extraocular Recovery in 143 Patients with Sarcoid Uveitis. *J. Clin. Med.* **2020**,

139. Giorgiutti, S.; Jamilloux, Y.; Gerfaud-Valentin, M.; Bert, A.; Ballonzoli, L.; Kodjikian, L.; Korganow, A.S.; Poindron, V.; Sève, P. The Course of Non-Infectious Uveitis in Pregnancy: A retrospective study of 79 pregnancies. *Graefes Arch. Clin. Exp. Ophthalmol.*

140. Sheppard JD, Toyos MM, Kempen JH, Kaur P, Foster CS. Difluprednate 0.05% versus prednisolone acetate 1% for endogenous anterior uveitis: a phase III, multicenter, randomized study. Invest Ophthalmol Vis Sci. 2014; 55(5):2993-3002. [PubMed: 24677110]

141. Rosenbaum JT, Choi D, Wilson DJ, Grossniklaus HE, Harrington CA, Sibley CH, Dailey RA, Ng JD, Steele EA, Czyz CN, Foster JA, Tse D, Alabiad C, Dubovy S, Parekh P, Harris GJ, Kazim M, Patel P, White V, Dolman P, Korn BS, Kikkawa D, Edward DP, Alkatan H, Al- Hussain H, Yeatts RP, Selva D, Stauffer P, Planck SR. Parallel Gene Expression Changes in Sarcoidosis Involving the Lacrimal Gland, Orbital Tissue, or Blood. JAMA Ophthalmol. 2015

142. Khurana RN, Porco TC. Efficacy and Safety of Dexamethasone Intravitreal Implant for Persistent Uveitic Cystoid Macular Edema. Retina. 2015

143. Ozkok A, Saleh OA, Sigford DK, Heroman JW, Schaal S. THE OMAR STUDY: Comparison of Ozurdex and Triamcinolone Acetonide for Refractory Cystoid Macular Edema in Retinal Vein Occlusion. Retina. 2015

144. Jaffe GJ, Martin D, Callanan D, Pearson PA, Levy B, ComstockT, Fluocinolone Acetonide Uveitis Study G. Fluocinolone acetonide implant (Retisert) for noninfectious posterior uveitis: thirty-four-week results of a multicenter randomized clinical study. Ophthalmology. 2006; 113(6): 1020-1027. [PubMed: 16690128]

145. Goldstein DA, Godfrey DG, Hall A, Callanan DG, Jaffe GJ, Pearson PA, Usner DW, ComstockTL. Intraocular pressure in patients with uveitis treated with fluocinolone acetonide implants. Arch Ophthalmol. 2007; 125(11):1478-1485. [PubMed: 17923537]

146. Multicenter Uveitis Steroid Treatment Trial Research G. Sugar EA, Holbrook JT, Kempen JH, Burke AE, Drye LT, Thorne JE, Louis TA, Jabs DA, Altaweel MM, Frick KD. Cost-effectiveness of fluocinolone acetonide implant versus systemic therapy for noninfectious intermediate, posterior, and panuveitis. Ophthalmology. 2014; 121(10):1855-1862. [PubMed: 24908205]

147. Dev S, McCallum RM, Jaffe GJ. Methotrexate treatment for sarcoid-associated panuveitis. Ophthalmology. 1999; 106(1):111-118. [PubMed: 9917790]

148. Bhat P, Cervantes-Castaneda RA, Doctor PP, Anzaar F, Foster CS. Mycophenolate mofetil therapy for sarcoidosis-associated uveitis. Ocul Immunol Inflamm. 2009; 17(3):185-190. [PubMed: 19585361]

149. Walton RC, Nussenblatt RB, Whitcup SM. Cyclosporine therapy for severe sight-threatening uveitis in children and adolescents. Ophthalmology. 1998; 105(11):2028-2034. [PubMed: 9818601]

150. Murphy CC, Greiner K, Plskova J, Duncan L, Frost NA, Forrester JV, Dick AD. Cyclosporine vs tacrolimus therapy for posterior and intermediate uveitis. Arch Ophthalmol. 2005; 123(5):634- 641 [PubMed: 15883282].

151. Jabs DA, Rosenbaum JT, Foster CS, Holland GN, Jaffe GJ, Louie JS, Nussenblatt RB, Stiehm ER, Tessler H, Van Gelder RN, Whitcup SM, Yocum D. Guidelines forthe use of immunosuppressive drugs in patients with ocular inflammatory disorders: recommendations of an expert panel. Am J Ophthalmol. 2000; 130(4):492-513. [PubMed: 11024423]

152. Gangaputra S, Newcomb CW, Liesegang TL, Kacmaz RO, Jabs DA, Levy-Clarke GA, Nussenblatt RB, Rosenbaum JT, Suhler EB, Thorne JE, Foster CS, Kempen JH, Systemic Immunosuppressive Therapy for Eye Diseases Cohort S. Methotrexate for ocular inflammatory diseases.

Ophthalmology. 2009; 116(11):2188-2198. e2181. [PubMed: 19748676]

153. Daniel E, Thorne JE, Newcomb CW, Pujari SS, Kacmaz RO, Levy-Clarke GA, Nussenblatt RB, Rosenbaum JT, Suhler EB, Foster CS, Jabs DA, Kempen JH. Mycophenolate mofetil for ocular inflammation. Am J Ophthalmol. 2010; 149(3):423- 432. e421-422. [PubMed: 20042178]

154. Pasadhika S, Kempen JH, Newcomb CW, Liesegang TL, Pujari SS, Rosenbaum JT, Thorne JE, Foster CS, Jabs DA, Levy-Clarke GA, Nussenblatt RB, Suhler EB. Azathioprine for ocular inflammatory diseases. Am J Ophthalmol. 2009; 148(4):500- 509. e502. [PubMed: 19570522]

155. Kacmaz RO, Kempen JH, Newcomb C, Daniel E, Gangaputra S, Nussenblatt RB, Rosenbaum JT, Suhler EB, Thorne JE, Jabs DA, Levy-Clarke GA, Foster CS. Cyclosporine for ocular inflammatory diseases. Ophthalmology. 2010; 117(3):576-584. [PubMed: 20031223]

156. Jaffe GJ, Thorne JE, Scales D, Franco P, Tari SR, Camez A, Song AP, Kron M, BarisaniAsenbauer T, Dick AD. Adalimumab in patients with active, non-infectious uveitis requiring highdose corticosteroids: the VISUAL-1 trial. ARVO 2015 Annual Meeting Abstracts by Scientific Section/Group - Immunology/Microbiology. 2015:73- 74.

157. Suhler EB, Smith JR, Wertheim MS, Lauer AK, Kurz DE, Pickard TD, Rosenbaum JT. A prospective trial of infliximab therapy for refractory uveitis: preliminary safety and efficacy outcomes. Arch Ophthalmol. 2005; 123(7):903-912. [PubMed: 16009830]

158. Suhler EB, Smith JR, Giles TR, Lauer AK, Wertheim MS, Kurz DE, Kurz PA, Lim L, Mackensen F, Pickard TD, Rosenbaum JT. Infliximab therapy for refractory uveitis: 2- year results of a prospective trial. Arch Ophthalmol. 2009; 127(6):819-822. [PubMed: 19506209]

159. Pritchard C, Nadarajah K. Tumour necrosis factor alpha inhibitor treatment for sarcoidosis refractory to conventional treatments: a report of five patients. Ann Rheum Dis. 2004; 63(3):318- 320. [PubMed: 14962969]

160. Doty JD, Mazur JE, Judson MA. Treatment of sarcoidosis with infliximab. Chest. 2005; 127(3): 1064-1071. [PubMed: 15764796]

161. Benitez-del-Castillo JM, Martinez-de-la-Casa JM, Pato-Cour E, Mendez-Fernandez R, LopezAbad C, Matilla M, Garcia-Sanchez J. Long-term treatment of refractory posterior uveitis with anti-TNFalpha (infliximab). Eye (Lond). 2005; 19(8):841-845. [PubMed: 15389273]

162. Erckens RJ, Mostard RL, Wijnen PA, Schouten JS, Drent M. Adalimumab successful in sarcoidosis patients with refractory chronic non-infectious uveitis. Graefes Arch Clin Exp Ophthalmol. 2012; 250(5):713-720 [PubMed: 22119879]

163. Smith JA, Thompson DJ, Whitcup SM, Suhler E, Clarke G, Smith S, Robinson M, Kim J, Barron KS. A randomized, placebo-controlled, double-masked clinical trial of etanercept for the treatment of uveitis associated with juvenile idiopathic arthritis. Arthritis Rheum. 2005; 53(1):18-23. [PubMed: 15696578]

164. Baughman RP, Lower EE, Bradley DA, Raymond LA, Kaufman A. Etanercept for refractory ocular sarcoidosis: results of a double-blind randomized trial. Chest. 2005; 128(2):1062-1047. [PubMed: 16100213]

165. William M, Faez S, Papaliodis GN, Lobo AM. Golimumab for the treatment of refractory juvenile idiopathic arthritis-associated uveitis. J Ophthalmic Inflamm Infect. 2012; 2(4):231-233. [PubMed: 22581347]

166. Cordero-Coma M, Calvo-Rio V, Adan A, Blanco R, Alvarez-Castro C, Mesquida M, Calleja S, Gonzalez-Gay MA, Ruiz de Morales JG. Golimumab as rescue therapy for refractory immunemediated uveitis: a three-center experience. Mediators Inflamm. 2014; 2014:717598. [PubMed: 24976689]

167. Calvo-Rio V, de la Hera D, Blanco R, Beltran-Catalan E, Loricera J, Canal J, Ventosa J, Cifrian JM, Ortiz-Sanjuan F, Rueda-Gotor J, Gonzalez-Vela MC, Gonzalez- Lopez M, Gonzalez-Gay MA. Golimumab in uveitis previously treated with other anti- TNF-alpha drugs: a retrospective study of three cases from a single center and literature review. Clin Exp Rheumatol. 2014; 32(6): 864-868. [PubMed: 25288110]

168. Izzi S, Francesconi F, Visca P, Altieri A, De Mutiis C, Trevisan G, Bonifati C. Pulmonary sarcoidosis in a patient with psoriatic arthritis during infliximab therapy. Dermatol Online J. 2010; 16(5):16. [PubMed: 20492833]

169. Clementine RR, Lyman J, Zakem J, Mallepalli J, Lindsey S, Quinet R. Tumor necrosis factoralpha antagonist-induced sarcoidosis. J Clin Rheumatol. 2010; 16(6):274-279. [PubMed: 20808167]

170. Daien CI, Monnier A, Claudepierre P, Constantin A, Eschard JP, Houvenagel E, Samimi M, Pavy S, Pertuiset E, Toussirot E, Combe B, Morel J, Club Rhumatismes et I. Sarcoid-like granulomatosis in patients treated with tumor necrosis factor blockers: 10 cases. Rheumatology
(Oxford). 2009; 48(8):883-886. [PubMed: 19423648]

171. Dhaille F, Viseux V, Caudron A, Dadban A, Tribout C, Boumier P, Clabaut A, Lok C. Cutaneous sarcoidosis occurring during anti-TNF-alpha treatment: report of two cases. Dermatology. 2010; 220(3):234-237. [PubMed: 20185892]

172. Metyas SK, Tadros RM, Arkfeld DG. Adalimumab-induced noncaseating granuloma in the bone marrow of a patient being treated for rheumatoid arthritis. Rheumatol Int. 2009; 29(4):437-439. [PubMed: 18762943]

173. Moisseiev E, Shulman S. Certolizumab-induced uveitis: a case report and review of the literature. Case Rep Ophthalmol. 2014; 5(1):54-59. [PubMed: 24707273]

174. Takase H, *et al.* Recommendations for the management of ocular sarcoidosis from the International Workshop on Ocular Sarcoidosis, *BrJ Ophthalmol* 2021;. doi:10.1136/bjophthalmol-2020-317354

175. Suhler EB, Lim LL, Beardsley RM, Giles TR, Pasadhika S, Lee ST, de Saint Sardos A, Butler NJ, Smith JR, Rosenbaum JT. Rituximab therapy for refractory scleritis: results of a phase I/II doseranging, randomized, clinical trial. Ophthalmology. 2014; 121(10):1885-1891. [PubMed: 24953794]

176. Huddleston SM, Houser KH, Walton RC. Thalidomide for recalcitrant nodular scleritis in sarcoidosis. JAMA Ophthalmol. 2014; 132(11):1377-1379. [PubMed: 25078792]

177. Brownstein S, Liszauer AD, Carey WD, Nicolle DA. Sarcoidosis of the eyelid skin. Can J Ophthalmol. 1990; 25(5):256-259. [PubMed: 2207873]

178. Oh JY, Wee WR. Cyclosporine for conjunctival sarcoidosis. Ophthalmology. 2008; 115(1):222. [PubMed: 18166429]

179. Akpek EK, Ilhan-Sarac O, Green WR. Topical cyclosporin in the treatment of chronic sarcoidosis of the conjunctiva. Arch Ophthalmol. 2003;

180. Pasadhika S, Smith JR. Treatment of uveitic macular edema: an overview and update. Ophthalmology International. 2008:97-103. Spring.

181. Cordero Coma M, Sobrin L, Onal S, Christen W, Foster CS. Intravitreal bevacizumab for treatment of uveitic macular edema. Ophthalmology. 2007;

182. Acharya NR, Hong KC, Lee SM. Ranibizumab for refractory uveitis-related macular edema. Am J Ophthalmol. 2009;

183. Edelsten C, Pearson A, Joynes E, Stanford MR, Graham EM. The ocular and systemic prognosis of patients presenting with sarcoid uveitis. Eye (Lond). 1999;

184. Karma A, Huhti E, Poukkula A. Course and outcome of ocular sarcoidosis. Am J Ophthalmol. 1988;

185. Ossewaarde-van Norel J, Ten Dam-van Loon N, de BoerJH, Rothova A. Long- term visual prognosis of peripheral multifocal chorioretinitis. Am J Ophthalmol. 2015

Table of contents

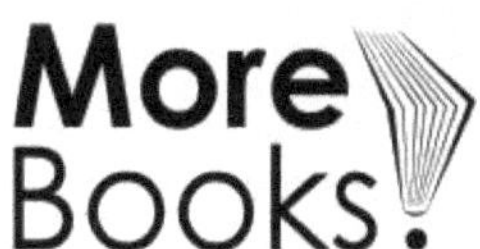

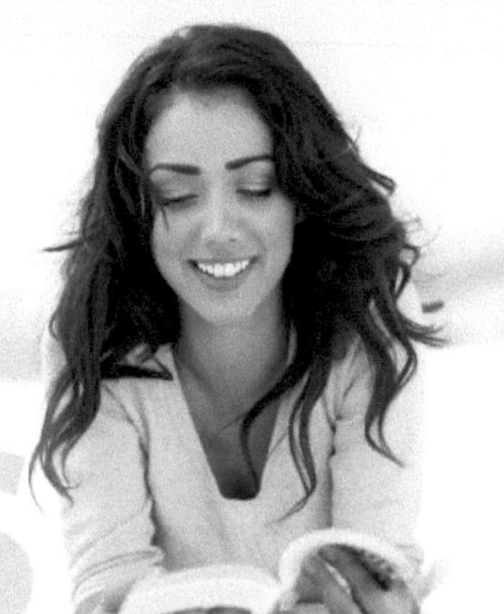

yes I want morebooks!

Buy your books fast and straightforward online - at one of world's fastest growing online book stores! Environmentally sound due to Print-on-Demand technologies.

Buy your books online at
www.morebooks.shop

Kaufen Sie Ihre Bücher schnell und unkompliziert online – auf einer der am schnellsten wachsenden Buchhandelsplattformen weltweit! Dank Print-On-Demand umwelt- und ressourcenschonend produzi ert.

Bücher schneller online kaufen
www.morebooks.shop

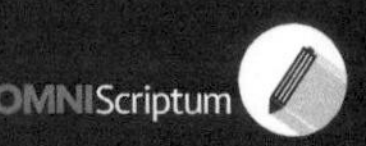